BUMS TUMS & BINGO WINGS

Karl Henry is one Ireland's leading personal trainers, well known for his work on TV's *Operation Transformation* and responsible for creating some of the most famous physiques in fashion, music, politics and industry.

He holds a BSc (hons) Sports Management from University College Dublin along with personal training qualifications, and is currently studying for an exercise and nutrition masters science degree.

Karl has a weekly health column in the *Irish Daily Mail*, and is regular contributor to TV and radio on health matters.

As well as his personal training and media work, he regularly lectures on fitness and wellbeing, and is a self-described fitness fanatic, each year finding a new sport to further his knowledge to pass on to his clients. His interests include hill-walking, cycling, triathlon, swimming, mountain biking, kite surfing, surfing, marathons, ironman triathlons and, more recently, ultra-marathons.

BUMS TUMS & BINGO WINGS

The Four-step Plan
TO A
FIT, FIRM, FABULOUS
NEW YOU

KARL HENRY

HACHETTE
BOOKS
IRELAND

First published in 2013 by Hachette Books Ireland
A division of Hachette UK Ltd.

Copyright © 2013 Karl Henry

A CIP catalogue record for this title is available from the British Library.

ISBN 978 14447 4346 3

Typeset and layout design by redrattledesign.com
Cover design by cabinlondon.co.uk
Cover photo by Partick Bolger

Printed and bound by CPI Group (UK) Ltd, Croydon, CR0 4YY

Hachette Books Ireland policy is to use papers that are natural, renewable and recyclable products and made from wood grown in sustainable forests. The logging and manufacturing processes are expected to conform to the environmental regulations of the country of origin.

Slightly altered versions of Appendices 1 & 2 originally featured in Karl's *Irish Daily Mail* 'Good Health' column, and are reproduced here with their kind permission.

Hachette Books Ireland
8 Castlecourt Centre
Castleknock
Dublin 15, Ireland

A division of Hachette UK Ltd
338 Euston Road
London NW1 3BH
www.hachette.ie

To my Mum, Dad and brother Cathal,
thank you for encouraging me to dream and
to believe that with hard work those
dreams can come true.

Acknowledgements

To Jean, thank you for sharing in my dreams and for supporting me no matter what crazy idea I come up with.

To Noel and Niamh at NK management, without you both these dreams wouldn't come true.

To Breda Purdue, Ciara Considine at all at Hachette Books Ireland, thank you for believing in this idea and doing such a great job.

To Regina and Gillian at the *Irish Daily Mail*, thank you for helping me to write weekly on what I believe in.

To Philip, Steve, Niamh and everyone at VIP & RTÉ, thank you for your support and belief.

To my clients – what can I say? Your hard work and results give meaning to what I do, you are all an inspiration.

To those who buy the book, thank you for believing in what I do. These pages will give you the tools to change your body and your thinking about health and your life. All my experience is contained here, and my clients results are testimony to just how well this plan works. Now it's your turn to get those results. Good luck, and don't forget to email me with your progress!

CONTENTS

INTRODUCTION

WHAT THE BTBW PLAN WILL DO FOR YOU

My name is Karl Henry. I am a personal trainer – though I am not a Lycra-clad, beefed-up bully who has always been ripped and super-fit and who can't understand why you are not super-fit too.

I was the last on the laps when I was in school, and it was only in my twenties that I started to take my fitness seriously – building it up slowly. Now, in my thirties, through hard work, perseverance and, it must be said, a taste for extreme sports, I have pushed my body to its limits, from ironmans to hundred-mile ultra marathons.

Through my own journey into fitness and my daily work with a huge range of clients, all with different backgrounds and needs, I have gained valuable insight into not only how to transform your own relationship with exercise and food, but also, how to sustain health and fitness for life. And that is exactly what I am setting out to help you do in the pages of this book.

I can teach you all you need to know to shape up, get fit and get the results you have always wanted. If you're sick of trying those fad diets that don't work, or fed up paying that monthly gym subscription that you never use, this book is here to help. If you've dreamed of going on holidays and actually wearing a bikini with confidence rather than covering up every ounce of flesh, then this book is tailor-made for you. My aim for you is to take up the Bums, Tums and Bingo Wings (BTBW) Plan and start to feel proud of your body and how you look. If you follow this plan, you will watch your body take on a new shape – it won't happen overnight, and it will take hard work, but it does happen, and quicker than you might think, through a sustainable plan that will soon have you walking down the street with that confident stride of someone who feels sexy in their own skin. Which is nothing less than what you deserve.

In the coming chapters, I can promise you this:

- There will be no off-putting Latin or scientific terms to confuse you

- The word 'diet' will take on a whole new meaning

- I will take all the confusion away and make getting fit and losing weight easy.

The reality is that getting in shape, losing weight and getting motivated is easy. Seriously, it is. Not easy in the January quick-fix way, I'm not trying to sell you something that will only last in the short term. I want to help you be the best you can be, not comparing you to anyone else. I will give you the tools to make weight loss, weight maintenance and long-term health easy, in a healthy way that will make the weight stay off long term. No milkshake meal replacements, no cabbage soup and no drill sergeant trying to belittle you by pumping up his own ego.

THE POKE TEST

Straighten your left arm down by your side, now take your right index finger and press it into your arm. See how much it travels – this is going to change over the coming weeks, you will see it travelling less and less as you firm up and your body fat drops.

Many women might dream of having Pippa Middleton's bum, but let's face it, it's hers and she's keeping it! But what every woman I've worked with wants without a doubt is to get their body into the best shape it can be in: sexy, firm and toned. You want to walk down the street beaming with health and wellbeing – does that sound like it would feel good? In this book, I will be guiding you through the minefield that is weight loss and showing you how to get your body into the best shape it has ever been in, getting you to the point that you walk down the street feeling like a million dollars!

Bums, tums and bingo wings are four words that strike dread into women right across the land. These are the areas that tend to be covered up and

FOOD FOR FITNESS

Believe it or not, 60 per cent of the success of a good fitness plan is about what food you eat – all the working out in the world won't make too much of a difference if you don't change your eating habits.

forgotten about! Well, I'm here to tell you that the time for covering up is over! This year you are going to be showing off your body with pride. There is no greater feeling than setting a goal, working hard for it and then being proud of the results. And that is exactly what is going to happen to you.

So what makes this book different to all the others, I hear you ask?

Simple.

. . . .

With this book, you will learn how to stay fit and slim long term. Not just for that wedding or holiday, but for many years to come.

. . . .

I will be telling you to have treat days where you can eat whatever you want – pizza, takeaway, whatever food you love to eat! You will have rest days where I want you to do no exercise at all, just sit back and let your body recover – sounds good, doesn't it? You will need to work hard at the exercises, no doubt about it, but they are doable. I won't let you do anything that is too complicated or too hard to follow. And there are three levels that you can move into from level 1, depending on your current fitness. By the time you reach level 3, you will be more than able for it!

An integral part of the BTBW Plan is proper eating. Fitness and health rely on each other: you can't have one without the other, not if you want real and lasting results. With this plan, you will be making changes to what you eat, maybe a little, maybe a lot, depending on your current diet.

I can promise you this: I won't be recommending any shakes or strange breakfasts, I won't be ruling out carbs or outlawing wine, and I won't be recommending any supplements that you have to spend money on. I will simply be showing you what you should and shouldn't eat, in plain English. Most importantly of all, I will be telling you why. Knowledge is power when it comes to health. The more you know, the more power you have over the choices you make.

I'll show you how to read a food label quickly, how to measure your fitness levels for free and what drinks you really should avoid.

BTBW IN FOUR EASY STEPS

 1. MOTIVATION

2. DIET

3. CARDIOVASCULAR EXERCISE
(the type that gets the heart pumping,
i.e. burning calories)

4. TARGETED BTBW EXERCISES.

It really is that simple. I'm not saying there isn't effort involved, or that the BTBW Plan won't challenge you – all change in life comes with challenge, that's what makes it worth it. But, trust me, if you follow each step in this book, you'll be more than happy to rise to the challenge, and it really will be straightforward.

I will break everything down for you into simple steps and then, over four weeks, you can watch your body change. Feel those jeans get looser until they are too big and you have to go out shopping for new ones. Watch your skin glow with radiance. Reduce the effects of PMS or the menopause.

You will also begin to sleep better and have more energy during the day.

I am lucky enough to see these changes on a day-to-day basis with my clients; now I want to share everything I know with you, so that you can see these changes for yourself, feel these changes and be proud of what you have achieved. This book is really about being the best that you can be. Not like some celebrity who has access to a personal trainer every day and who has a chef to cook for them. You are a busy person with a busy life. You work hard. You want to look your best and that is exactly what this book will help you do. So chin up, pen to the ready and let's start you on your journey to changing your life.

1

GETTING MOTIVATED THE BTBW WAY

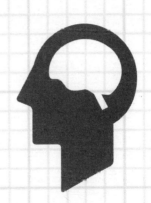

'It's not always easy. There are days when I feel like I'd murder a slice of chocolate cake, but what keeps me motivated is that picture in my head of the aubergine halter neck, fitted-waist bridesmaid dress and running across the finish line in Longford (not in the dress!) at a time of 1 hour 59 minutes and 59 seconds. And I realise that if I really want the chocolate cake, I can have it on Saturday as my treat.' – Sandra

Do you ever sit and wonder why you can't get off the couch and get in shape?

Do you admire other people who seem to be able to do it effortlessly? Yet, no matter how much you think you want to get in shape, you just seem unable to move.

Have you ever done a few weeks of training, then become bored or disillusioned and stopped? Wondered why?

WRITE IT DOWN

The reality is that someone with a plan will run rings around someone who doesn't have one. Get a pen and paper, and let's get going!

It all comes down to goal-setting, a key tool in motivating yourself.

Set aside a little time before you start to really look at the why and how of achieving your goals because this will pay huge dividends in the long run. It can be surprisingly tough to sit and think, but it really is an important step. Do you really think that Pippa got that bum by sitting on it? Yes, to some degree that bum is a result of genetics, but you can be sure that it's also the result of a planned approach to exercise – and diet.

And this type of planning is exactly what you need to bring to your exercise this year, next year and on into the future. Get your pen and paper ready, for here is your checklist to banish those motivational doubts for good.

FIVE KEY QUESTIONS

Getting motivated involves first getting straight with yourself. Being brutally honest at the outset will save you sure disappointment later. You are about to ask yourself five key questions, the answers to which will pave the way for a new you. Why? When? Where? Who? How? Look yourself straight in the eye now!

1: WHY?

Write whatever comes into your mind in terms of why you want to get fit. You may have to dig a little to discover the real reason, but without this reason – the true, honest reason – you will struggle. Maybe not initially, because you will be full of the endorphin rush that comes with exercise, the happy hormones that make you feel so good, but after a few weeks, your motivation will begin to wane. This is exactly what happens in February every year after the resolutions have been forgotten.

Think of where you are at this moment in time. Forget about judging yourself, try to step outside the arena of self-criticism and accept that you are where you are, full stop. From that perspective, ask yourself how you got to this point. What caused you to be at the fitness level you are at now? Was it progressive or recent? Are you happy about it? If not, why? How is it impacting on your quality of life? Ask yourself what it is that you really want to change. Once you discover this, you will really know why you want to start to get fit. Then, every time you struggle to get off the couch to go training, this thought will remind you why you're doing it, and you will overcome the obstacles that are standing in your way. I know it can be tough, but this little bit of soul-searching is the key to you looking your best.

YOUR MISSION STATEMENT

Take a few minutes to fill out the mission statement on the next page of this book. Keep it short and to the point. When you have done it, cut it out and stick it somewhere you will see it every day. As you start to achieve your goals, your mission statement may change as you set new ones. Update it and look at it every day. This will remind you of why you are here.

Sample mission statement:

I want to improve my fitness so that I can run around the park with the kids and not get out of breath. So that I can feel good in my skin again, and wear the clothes I want to wear. So that I can look super at Amanda's wedding in a dress that bares my arms. So that I can improve my tiredness levels that stop me moving from the couch in the evenings. I want to feel good about myself again and not cringe when I catch my reflection in a shop window. I aim to do this by following the BTBW Plan for life – I know this is not a quick fix.

MY MISSION STATEMENT

_____
_____
_____
_____
_____
_____
_____
_____
_____
_____
_____
_____
_____
_____
_____
_____
_____

Or

I've been working too hard at the expense of my own wellbeing. I want to create a better work-life balance and feel fit again. I want to lose the extra [fill in number] stone I know I'm carrying and wear the clothes I like, clothes that show off my curves instead of hiding my flab. I want to take care of my diet again and make time for proper eating, not takeaways and sugary carbs. By summer, I want to head off on holidays feeing confident about my beach body, instead of fixating about everyone else's! I want to find the old me again, who walked down the street with a spring in her step. I aim to do this by following the BTBW Plan for life – I know this is not a quick fix.

2: WHEN?

Now you know the why, you need to be definitive and concise. The less structured your plan, the more stuff is liable to get in the way. You need to prioritise for yourself, so the first thing to do is to make a start date and put it in your diary. Nothing comes in the way of this date! By making this time your priority, you will be investing it with the importance it deserves: this is *your* time. You should schedule forward your cardio workouts and exercise – which we'll come to later – too, because this ensures that you keep prioritising it, and makes it much more likely that you till stick to it. Initially you may feel guilty about giving yourself this time, but after two weeks, those diary entries will be sacrosanct to you.

The information that follows in this book will enable you to tailor your fitness routine to your needs at a given moment, but as a rule of thumb I recommend that anyone starting out on the BTBW Plan creates time for three one-hour sessions a week to devote to both cardiovascular exercise and your specific BTBW exercises. Over time, the intensity of the exercise changes in line with your increasing fitness, but the time dedicated to it remains fairly static.

People lead busy lives, it's true, but it's easy to convince ourselves that we don't have the time to devote to exercise or proper eating. Making time can mean prioritising, even leaving something else behind – but that something else could as easily be less time sitting on the couch with remote in hand, or 30 extra minutes in bed in the mornings. Getting out of bed 30 minutes earlier than usual, before the mayhem of the day has begun, and starting your BTBW routine will set you up for the day like nothing else, believe it!

3: WHERE?

Location is of key importance. If you're going to carry out your BTBW Plan in a gym, you need to feel that you are getting service and feel comfortable in the gym space. Ideally it should be somewhere close to your work or home, for ease of access. The farther away and more out of your everyday route it is, the harder it will be for you to get there, and the easier it will be to make excuses to avoid going. So choose carefully and put plenty of thought into it.

As we will go into shortly, cardiovascular exercise is a cornerstone of the BTBW routine. If you are going to be walking or running, then make sure you are going somewhere that is accessible and somewhere you like – the more you like the place, the more likely you are to go. Also, obviously, your personal safety should be taken into account. Remember, enjoyment is so important in every aspect of your fitness plan: the more you enjoy it, the longer you will keep it up.

4: WHO?

One of the most important questions I ask all my clients is: 'Who are you doing this for?' If the answer is anyone else but yourself, you need to think about that. Be honest with yourself. Because the truth is, unless you are taking up the BTBW Plan for yourself, chances are you won't reap the rewards that you should. Remember, you are the one who will be putting in the effort – and reaping the rewards! It's about you first, so never lose sight of that.

. . . .

It is no good trying to get fit to please someone else in your life, or live up to another person's ideal about how you should be, it has to come from within.

. . . .

Because when it gets tough and you get sore, you can be sure that you will struggle to keep going. But when you yourself are the primary reason, you dig deeper, work harder and stick to the plan. If you make an agreement with yourself not to give up, you will stick to that, because when you hit that 'wall', you know exactly why you are there and for whom you are making the effort. This can often be one of the hardest things to admit, to really admit to yourself that you are the one who wants to change but, tough as it may be, it is really important for you to succeed.

Inevitably, if you change because you think others will prefer you that way, you will be disappointed. After the initial compliments, life will resume as normal – unless you have made the change within. When you make the change within, then everything around you starts to change with it. So why not? Don't you deserve to be your best self – for yourself?

ONE STEP AT A TIME

Don't look at the mountain, look at the ground beneath your feet. That way you will avoid getting scared by the bigger picture. Think of the BTBW Plan in four-week segments. A lot can and will happen in that time. And when those segments begin to add up, the bigger picture – and summit – will take care of itself.

5: HOW?

What do you actually need to achieve your goal? Is it going to cost any money? Will it take much time out of your week? Try to complete a full analysis of the logistics of what you are going to do before you start, so that you can be confident that you can carry out your BTBW Plan without added stress.

Soon we will go into the specifics of the BTBW exercise routine, and depending on the results of the fitness tests that you will carry out on yourself, I will give you specific guidance on your tailored plan, including how much time to set aside to begin with, and how to build on that. You can then create your own personal regime.

Take the time now to write down the where, when and how of it, and aim to review these every time you achieve your goals and start a new phase of your plan. It's a foolproof but tough way to ensure that you are doing something for the right reasons. It can be hard to dig for the why, but once you find it, it will become the key to your long-term health!

Writing down your plan is the part many people don't do and it's also the reason why many people fall off the wagon or stop exercising. Goal-setting and planning are two underlying tools used by all successful people, whether they are dealing with weight loss or business; all the success stories will include these two elements somewhere, something that in my opinion we should all learn from and use in our own day-to-day lives.

So, what should be your goal for the first four weeks? What can you really achieve if you stick to the food and exercise plan? If you work hard and absorb all that I am going to tell you, I can promise you that you will:

WHEN?

WHERE?

WHO?

HOW?

- Begin to notice a discernible difference in the key areas of focus for the routine – your bum, your tum and your upper arms. And the muscle groups involved will be becoming much stronger which brings effects to all aspects of your body, from your back to your neck, shoulders and legs.

- Experience weight loss. Your digestion will be healthier too as your body has eliminated a lot of toxins from the new dietary changes and is now working much more efficiently.

- Feel more energetic, sleep better and experience more consistent good moods. You will learn to love those endorphins!

Below is a list of actual results that clients of mine have achieved, to show you what is possible in just four weeks:

- Lose ten pounds in weight.

- Lose four inches from your waist.

- Lose two inches from your legs.

- Have a firmer, tighter, higher bum!

THE BTBW Plan SAYS: Keep mum! The more people you tell about your plan, the harder it will be to achieve. While friends and work colleagues may mean the best for you, the pressure of knowing they are watching you will actually make it harder. Some may even try to demotivate you because they are envious of your motivation. Why not just work hard, get the results and let them tell you how great you look? This acts as one of the ultimate motivators because they didn't know you were training in the first place.

- Lose one inch from your arms.

- Have a resting heart rate that's five beats lower.

- Have more energy, less stress and more confidence.

- Have glowing skin that will make you the envy of all your friends.

Motivated yet?
You should be!

THE POWER OF REWARD

The fun part of setting goals is setting the reward you will give yourself when you achieve the goal. I'm not suggesting that you reward yourself with a big pizza, but whatever motivates you is fine by me (as long as it doesn't undo the good you've achieved!). The reward will help you to get up off the couch on those days when you're not really in the mood, because you know that if you don't get up and do it you may not get that reward.

For me, books are a great reward. I love to read, so if I am setting out a hard training block, I will set aside some reward goals every two or three weeks. These are short term and make it easier to stay focused and work as hard as I possibly can. Once I get the training done, I take my reward. Easy and functional, reward is one of the key elements of motivation that so many people forget about. It's nice to treat yourself, isn't it? Especially when you have worked so hard for it.

One method that I use with my clients involves clothes. Go in to your favourite clothes shop and try on a dress or top that doesn't fit quite right. Now go away and work your ass off for the four weeks, then go back to that shop, try the same item of clothing on and watch that smile widen on your face as you realise it now fits you perfectly. That change hasn't come as a result of nothing, you have worked hard for it, and that just increases the sense of satisfaction!

Enjoy your reward time, enjoy the feeling of pride as you get it and then use that feeling as a motivator for your next goal-setting journey.

FALLING OFF THE WAGON

So what happens if, despite your best intentions, you fall off the wagon? Something comes up that totally throws you, you miss one day of your BTBW Plan, one slips into two, and before you know it, you're back to your old ways.

Firstly, don't panic. Take a deep breath, let some of the stress and anguish out and take a look at what happened. Life isn't perfect and it doesn't always go to plan, don't beat yourself up about it. Just take a step outside any critical voice that's in your head, and try to understand what happened. Did you try to do too much too soon? Did you try a sport that, deep down, you knew you wouldn't like?

Once you realise why it didn't work, it's time to put together a new plan of attack.

. . . .

Failure is only a negative if you choose it to be.

. . . .

I have 'failed' at various endeavours on my journey to peak fitness, and each time I've learned so much about my training and my own body. My failures have given me invaluable knowledge that I wouldn't have learned if I had not tried the events that led to them. I simply used this information to improve my training for the next event – and you need to do exactly the same. Set a new goal, build a better plan, learn from the mistakes from the first plan and start working towards that goal.

I'd like to try an exercise now. Get a pen and paper, and imagine I am sitting in front of you and am going to train you for the next four weeks. You've done the when, where, who and why. Now comes the what. What would you like to achieve in that time?

A dress size down?

A decrease in inches?

Set those fantastic goals and then let's take a look at how you are going to achieve them.

2

LOVE YOUR GRUB AND GET THIN: THE BTBW FOOD PLAN

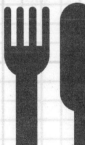

'My friends all ask what diet I'm on, but it never feels like a diet in the old-school sense. I've made small but sensible changes to my eating, making clever decisions so as to never feel hungry or bloated. My one treat day a week has become something I carefully consider, weigh up the pros and cons of every option and thoroughly enjoy it, guilt-free!' – Sandra

In this chapter, I am not going to give you a magic quick fix that will claim to change your body shape in five days. And, happily, there won't be a high-protein solution that will make your breath stink and take all the moisture out of your skin. Nor will there be a plan that will only make you heavier in the long term – like pretty much every quick fix on the market. What I will give you is everything you will ever need to know to be able to lose weight, lose body fat and gain more energy than ever before, in a lasting way. Because what we are going to create is a food plan for life that can apply equally to you as to anyone else you cook for, including kids!

I am also going to give you the knowledge behind what I tell you, because the more you know, the more control you have over the choices you make. I advocate a 'low GI' style of eating, which will:

- Improve your energy levels

- Improve your skin, hair and nails

- Help you lose weight

- Make you less likely to snack

- Lower your blood pressure, your cholesterol and your diabetes risk

- Improve how you deal with stress and work pressure

- Decrease negative side-effects of your menstrual cycle by balancing hormones

- Improve your motivation levels.

GI stands for glycaemic index, which is the measurement of glucose level increase in your blood from the food that you eat. Of all the different nutrient groups in food, carbohydrates are the highest on the GI, and refined carbohydrates are the worst offenders. Understanding the GI level of foods is central to the BTBW Food Plan.

I have eaten this type of diet for several years and all of my clients eat this way too. The results

I have got with this style of eating are incredible. From a weight perspective, you can easily lose up to a stone in six weeks. You will be firmer and more toned from your exercises, and, more importantly, you will be healthier. What's the point of being slim if you are not healthy?

As I've said, if you want to get proper results, fast, then your food is 60 per cent of the work! All the training in the world won't make the slightest bit of difference if you aren't eating healthily. The better your food, the better the results you will get.

THE BTBW FOOD PLAN ♥ LOW GI

So how does it apply to this new diet? As mentioned, GI is simply about the reaction of the sugar in your blood to the food that you eat. Some foods cause a high reaction in blood sugar, some a low reaction. The best diet is one low in GI. That's pretty much the basis of it.

Foods that have a high GI trigger a greater insulin response from your liver, which can promote fat storage in your body once your glycogen (energy converted from glucose) stores are full. High GI foods also cause a surge of energy that is followed by low blood sugar two or three hours later. This explains why your body craves more high-sugar foods a few hours after you have eaten them. You know that 11 o'clock break? Well that's exactly why it happens. You get trapped in this sugar cycle and that is one of the major causes of weight gain. High GI foods are high in sugar, usually of a refined kind, which is nutritionally low with no long-term health benefits, i.e. to be avoided.

. . . .

Low GI foods, on the other hand, cause a gradual increase in energy that sustains over a longer time frame. Your body uses more of the energy from these foods and stores less as fat.

. . . .

You will feel fuller for longer, have fewer cravings and more energy. So not only will a low GI diet help you lose weight, it will also give you more energy. It's a win-win situation!

A low GI diet has nothing to do with 'carb-cutting', a protein-based diet technique I don't recommend. But it has got to do with replacing what we'll call 'bad carbs' – high GI, low nutritional value – for good ones – low GI, high nutritional value. The ethos of a low GI diet is about eating unrefined, natural food of an unprocessed kind. The more processed a food, the more the nutritional value is compromised, and the greater tendency there is for additives. Unprocessed food is closer

THE GREAT DIET MYTH

Products marketed as 'fat-free', 'low-cal' and 'diet' more often than not are higher in preservatives, additives and artificial flavourings than the products they are replacing. They have no place in the BTBW Food Plan. The good news is that you will be eating the foods you like to eat, just with some variation. A healthy diet is not about starvation, it's about loving food and feeling its benefits. Get ready to change your ideas about food, and wake up to just how good it can be – and healthy. And you won't need to pick up a single fat-free or diet product off the supermarket shelf. You can bin those right along with the diet myths you have in your head, reinforced possibly from years of yo-yo dieting. Replace them with this proven truth: A DELICIOUS DIET CAN ALSO BE A WEIGHT-LOSS DIET. Read on, it's all about to become clear.

to how nature intended, and therefore easier for your body to digest and benefit from.

In the pages that follow you will develop the knowledge you need to recognise what foods will deliver what type of energy and also which foods will promote weight loss and which will cause weight gain.

The first thing you'll need to address in the BTBW Food Plan is your larder. You will be making some basic replacements – don't worry about throwing everything out and running out to the shops. But do replace as you go, and aim to make the changes as swiftly as you can. This new larder will be a low GI one, with a whole lot less sugar weighing it down.

We'll go into more detail shortly on the exact foods you should be eating, but below is a quick swap list with some of the more common foods that form part of our daily diet.

HIGH GI	LOW GI
White bread	Brown bread
White rice	Brown rice
White pasta	Brown pasta
Special K and other refined cereals	All Bran/Bran Flakes/ Porridge

Fizzy drinks	Water
Flavoured water	Water with diced fruit
Potatoes	Sweet potatoes
Cream-based sauces	Tomato-based sauces
Creamy dressings	Oil-based dressings

Those are just some obvious food types, but it shows that by making easy choices, you can change the GI content of the food you are eating.

As mentioned, all foods have a GI number, and for the BTBW Food Plan we should be aiming to eat foods whose number is 55 or lower. Below is information on some of the main foods we regularly eat:

GI RATING			
Potato (baked)	95	Carrots cooked	85
Potato (chips)	95	Corn flakes	85
Puffed rice	95	Popcorn	85
Mashed potato	90	White bread	85
Rice pre-cooked	90	Rice cakes	85
Honey (don't forget this is a natural sugar)	90	Potato crisps	80
Baked beans (cooked)	80	Melon	65
Tapioca	80	Banana	65

White crackers	80	Processed orange juice	65
Pumpkin	75	Raisins	65
White baguettes	75	Shortbread biscuits	55
Watermelon	72	Petit beurre biscuits	55
Unprocessed white bread	70	White pasta	55
Cereals (sugared)	70	Unrefined (unprocessed) flour	55
Chocolate bars	70	Buckwheat	50
Potato (peeled and boiled)	70	Pancakes	50
Sugar	70	Sweet potato	50
Turnip	70	Kiwi fruit	50
Cornflour	70	Basmati rice	50
Maize	70	Brown rice	50
Pre-cooked, non-stick rice	70	Sorbet	50
Soft drinks	70	Porridge	49
White noodles	70	Home-made brown bread	45
Processed brown bread	65	Brown pitta	43
Boiled potatoes	65	Peas	40
Semolina	65	Grapes	40
Fresh orange juice	40	Beans (haricot)	30
Fresh apple juice	40	Beans (French)	30
Rye bread	40	Brown lentils	30

Brown pasta	40	Cooked chickpeas	30
Kidney beans	40	Fruit preserve (without sugar)	30
Wholegrain bread	40	Dark chocolate	30
Corn on the cob	35	Green lentils	30
Quinoa (cooked)	35	Split peas	22
Peas-dried (cooked)	35	Cherries	22
Raw carrots	35	Plums	22
Full-milk yoghurt (plain)	35	Grapefruit	22
Skimmed-milk yoghurt (plain)	35	Fructose	22
Orange	35	Cooked soya	20
Pear	35	Peanuts	20
Fig	35	Apricots (fresh)	20
Apricots	35	Walnuts	20
Semi-skimmed milk	35	Onions	20
Soy milk	35	Garlic	15
Bran-based breakfast cereals	30	Green veg, lettuce, mushrooms	10
Peach	30	Tomatoes, aubergines, red peppers	10
Apple	30	Cabbage, broccoli	10
Note: Meats/fish are so low in carbohydrates that they have a GI rating of zero			

When shopping, you need to take this into consideration. Unfortunately, though, at this point in time, most food labels don't actually have GI numbers on them. This is starting to change, but it's still not a regular occurrence. So I am going to equip you with a simple tool to check how suitable foods you buy are to your BTBW Food Plan. You are essentially looking for one key ingredient when you look at a food label: sugar.

STANDING UP TO THE BULLY OF THE WAISTLINE

. . . .

Sugar has become the enemy of waistlines throughout the world, and its level of consumption in the diet has a massive impact on whether you put on – or lose – weight.

. . . .

The fat content of food is no longer the be all and end all. Good fats, which are called unsaturated fats, taken in moderation have positive health effects in the body. But the positive effects of sugar, and especially the refined kind which is typically added to processed foods to make them tasty to our sugar-sensitive palates, are few and far between. And refined sugar is in *all* high GI foods – so when it enters your bloodstream it will send your energy levels through the roof, triggering insulin production in your body and promoting fat storage. This is especially true in high doses, because as I've mentioned, once your carbohydrate stores are full, everything else is stored as fat. It's time to stand up to it – and fight to regain your waistline!

BYE BYE CELLULITE

Diets that are high in sugar also tend to be high in toxins, such as additives and preservatives, leading to increased cellulite in your body. From my experience with clients, the higher the sugar content in their diets, the higher the cellulite content in their bodies. Reducing the sugar intake and increasing the amount of water drunk can produce a dramatic difference in cellulite in just two weeks. Too much sugar also affects the skin, increasing its dryness and the occurrence of spots.

So from now on, I want you to look at the sugar content in the foods you are eating. Look at the food label on the back of the packet. Under carbohydrates you will see an 'of which sugars' value. The lower this value, the better the food. Ideally, aim to have a sugar content of less that 40 per cent of the carbohydrate value. So if there is 100g of carbohydrates on the label, ensure that there is less than 40g of sugar. It's as simple as that!

BYE BYE SUGAR-FREE

Many 'sugar-free' and 'diet' products are on the market catering to our sugar concerns, marketing themselves as an ideal substitute – all the taste without the negative effects. But if you're someone who has bought into this, I'm afraid I have some bad news for you. These products contain artificial sweeteners, the most common of which is called aspartame, which gives it that sweet taste you crave. Aspartame is sweeter than sugar (and cheaper) but, unfortunately, it's not the cure-all it purports to be. This is because, just like sugar, it can cause your body to produce insulin. And too much insulin production promotes fat storage. So although it may say 'diet' on the label, there is increasing evidence to show that it may have a similar effect in your body to sugar. For the BTBW Food Plan, 'diet' drinks and products are for the bin.

BYE BYE CALORIE-COUNTING

And even if aspartame can help you to lose weight as part of a calorie-controlled diet, the happy fact is that calorie-counting has no place in the BTBW Food Plan. Many of my clients are surprised to hear this, in fact some get nervous as it takes them out of their comfort zone. We've been trained to believe that the only way to lose weight is by counting calories. If we have to give that up, how will we know how to limit our eating?

What they quickly realise, though, is that letting go of calorie-counting is a liberation. Let's be honest – it's a pain in the ass, right? Life is for living, not adding up!

. . . .

The BTBW Food Plan is about eating healthy foods that you enjoy, until you feel satisfied, using the GI index as your

45

guide. No adding up necessary! It's about learning to read the body's signs as to when we've had enough food, by eating slowly and taking time to chew your food properly (which will also aid your digestion). It's about bringing the joy back into eating – and leaving the guilt behind. Remember, regular over-eating has nothing to do with loving food. There can be emotional and physical reasons, and one can feed into the other: we indulge our craving because we feel bad, only serving to reinforce our craving. The BTBW Food Plan is about breaking those habits down, gently and firmly. It's about loving your grub – and loving your life. Happily, these two things reinforce each other too, but in a positive way.

. . . .

Once you've cracked the GI index, that really is all you need to know to make the BTBW Food Plan a weight-loss certainty, and calorie-counting a thing of the past. It really can be done!

READ THE LABEL!

So let's take a look at the other aspects of food labels we need to take into consideration when stocking our BTBW Food Plan larder.

Energy:

This is the total energy content for whatever food you are eating. Energy is measured in kilojoules (kj) and kilocalories (kcal). The energy content on the label simply tells you the total amount of energy in that food. The recommended daily intake for the average woman is 1,800–2,000 calories – this is a useful guideline, but in realty it varies a lot depending on size, shape and levels of activity. And remember, the BTBW Food Plan is not based around calorie-counting!

Protein:

This is the nutrient in the diet that promotes growth and repair and is of key importance as part of a balanced diet. Each gram of protein you eat has four calories in it. Foods that are high in protein are meats, fish, eggs, tofu, Quorn (a vegetarian meat substitute), nuts and pulses (such as lentils). The recommended daily intake is 1–2 grams of protein per kilogram of body weight.

Carbohydrates:

These are your main energy source. Cut them out completely and you will be constantly tired. As we know, some carbohydrates are high GI and some are low GI. On the food label, the 'of which sugars' value is the one to look out for – ideally, it should be no more than and preferably less than 40% of the overall carbohydrate value.

THE 'NO MORE THAN 40%' RULE

In the absence of GI information on food labels, understanding the 'of which sugars' part of the carbohydrate information is vitally important. This is because the higher the sugar content as part of the overall carbohydrate total, the higher the GI rating for that food. So remember your BTBW rule of thumb: NO MORE THAN 40% OF OVERALL CARBOHYDRATE LEVEL – AND PREFERABLY LESS.

There are four calories per gram of carbohydrate that you eat. Carbohydrate recommendations vary depending on your activity levels, but I normally recommend 2–4 grams of carbohydrates per kilogram of body weight per day.

Fat:

Just as we've been trained to think that calorie-counting is necessary for weight loss, we've been trained to think that fat is the enemy of waistlines! And it's true that high fat foods eaten in excess will cause weight gain. But fats, and particularly what we'll call good fats, taken in proper quantities, are highly important in the diet and have excellent health benefits, including keeping your hair, skin and nails healthy.

There are three types of fat, the first, unsaturated, being the most friendly to the BTBW Food Plan:

- **Unsaturated fats:** These are found in plant foods and fish. In the right quantity, these promote a healthy heart.

- **Saturated fats:** These fats are found in meat and dairy products and are also in palm and coconut oils. Eating too much saturated fat can raise blood cholesterol levels and increase the risk of heart disease.

- **Trans fats:** Also often referred to as hydrogenated fats, these are often found in margarine, many snack foods such as biscuits, processed foods and takeaway foods. When you see 'hydrogenated' or 'partially hydrogenated' oils on an ingredient list, the food contains trans fats, which have been shown to raise levels of 'bad' (LDL) cholesterol, lower those of 'good' (HDL) cholesterol, and increase the risk of heart disease.[*]

The recommended daily allowance (RDA) is 65 grams of fat. Each gram of fat you eat contains nine calories.

Salt:
This is essential for your normal body functions, but too much of it will make your body hold on to fluid. So if you are prone to holding fluid, cut back on the salt! There is generally more than enough salt in the foods that we eat, so that you actually don't need table salt at all. The recommended daily allowance is six grams.

---

[*]New York City has been pioneering in its stance on trans fats, recognising their negative impact on health: they've been banned from restaurants there since 2006.

There are many other ingredients on a food label, but those listed above are the most important ones. Now when you go to the supermarket, take a little time and compare the labels of your favourite foods, because you will be amazed at the difference between foods. This is another step in gaining power over your food intake, another tool that you now possess to ensure that you are eating the best foods possible.

We will now look at some low GI foods that you can choose from, to show you exactly what you should be eating.

YOUR BTBW BREAKFAST

. . . .

Miss this at your peril! When you skip breakfast, your body slows down, burns fewer calories during the day and naturally stores more fat. This is the one meal that you really have to hit every day, giving your body the kick start it needs!

. . . .

As the food labels of most cereals testify, they are laden with sugar and salt, leading to a very high GI level. Below is my top list of breakfast-based foods that you can choose from:

- Low-sugar granola and natural yoghurt/ skimmed milk

- Brown bread toast with real butter

- Eggs in most forms (boiled, scrambled, poached or in an omelette)

- Fruit salad with natural yoghurt

- Low-fat yoghurt with honey

- Wholemeal or spelt flour pancakes

- Porridge with low-fat milk or water

- And, to drink, a large glass of water.

Sample meals:
- Bran flakes with skimmed milk

- Scrambled eggs with brown bread toast

- Wholemeal pancakes

- Porridge with skimmed milk and honey

- Mushroom and tomato omelette.

LUNCH

Now that you have got rid of your high GI breakfasts, you won't have sugar cravings at eleven o'clock like you used to – lunch will become something you look forward to, rather than something you crave. This is the time to refuel your body with a mixture of low GI carbohydrates and protein. Take your pick from the options below:

- Mixed salad with protein (e.g. meat, fish, eggs or tofu)

- Soup, preferably home-made but if buying a carton, read the label to make sure that it fits with your low GI plan – the 'no more than 40%' rule.

- Brown bread sandwich

- Wholegrain bagel with low GI filling

- Brown wrap with low GI filling

- Brown pitta bread with low GI filling.

Sample meals:

- Brown bread sandwich with turkey, lettuce and tomato

- Chicken salad with balsamic vinegar dressing

- Minestrone soup

- Wholegrain crackers with tuna

- Wholemeal wrap with peppers, onions and lettuce.

DINNER

Dinner should be another good, solid meal, with protein and vegetables – vegetables are a wonderfully nutrient-rich, naturally low GI food so essential to the BTBW Food Plan. Make sure to eat your greens, but keep it colourful too – the more you mix it up, the wider the range of nutrients you'll get. Brown carbs should form part of this meal too, but keep the portions low especially if it's later in the evening when you're sitting down to eat, as they take longer to digest. Take your pick from the list below:

- **Meat or vegetarian proteins:**

    Lean beef, chicken, turkey, fish, lamb, Quorn (a vegetarian meat substitute), tofu, nuts, lentils/beans.

- **Vegetables:**

    All vegetables are welcome but those higher in GI number, such as root vegetables (carrots, parsnips, squash), should be taken in moderation.
    Feel free to go wild on the lower GI ones, such as tomatoes, cucumber, artichokes, asparagus, peppers, celery, mushrooms, French beans, leeks, cabbage, cauliflower, gherkins, avocado, bean sprouts, watercress, lettuce, broccoli.

- **Carbohydrates:**

  Brown pasta, brown rice, wholemeal couscous, sweet potatoes.

Sample meals:

- Brown pasta with tomato-based sauce and chicken

- Beef stir fry with brown rice

- Grilled tofu kebabs with peppers and onions

- White fish and stir-fried vegetables

- Cajun chicken breasts with sweet potato fries.

SNACKS

For anyone trying to lose weight, snacking is an important thing to take into consideration. I recommend that you snack no more than twice a day. BTBW-friendly snack foods are:

- Small wholemeal scones, natural yoghurt (certain brands are naturally low in fat so, again, check the labels), nuts (handful), wholegrain Ryvita and cottage cheese, seeds, fruit.

Sample snacks:

- Fruit (no more than two per day)

- Handful of nuts

- Natural yoghurt and honey.

Fruits are a fantastic form of nutrients, but remember they contain relatively high levels of sugar. I would recommend limiting your fruit intake to around two pieces per day (or a handful of berries/grapes). Remember, for the BTBW Food Plan to work, moderation of sugar intake is key.

FLUIDS

Your body needs fluids during the day to stop it becoming dehydrated. All of the major bodily functions require water, and unbeknownst to us, many of us go through the day dehydrated. By drinking fluid regularly during the day, you will keep your body functioning properly and help it to eliminate waste, such as toxins and fat, too.

If you haven't drunk water regularly for quite some time, one of the instant effects of increased hydration will, unsurprisingly, be more trips to the loo, which is a great sign as it's your body regulating itself, excreting all the excess fluid and toxins that it was holding on to. This will settle down after a week or so to a more regular pattern as your body adjusts accordingly.

People often ask me if tea and coffee count as part of a daily fluid intake. The answer is, they are fluid, so literally speaking, yes they do. However, they are also diuretics, meaning they reduce the amount of water in the body, so for the purposes of the BTBW Food Plan we don't count them in our daily fluid intake.

THE POWER OF H^2O

There is nothing better than good old-fashioned water. Two litres is the normal recommendation unless you are highly active, in which case you may need to increase it. The easiest way of ensuring that you are drinking the right amount is to get a 2-litre bottle of water every morning and simply aim to have drunk the bottle by the end of the day – this takes away the guesswork and glass-counting. Avoid flavoured water because it has added sugar or sugar substitute, but if you find still water too plain, then you can chop up some pieces of fruit yourself (such as a lemon or an orange) and put this into the water to flavour it naturally.

For reasons of limiting sugar intake, fruit juices are also best avoided in general and, if being taken in moderation, freshly squeezed is best. Most juices you find on supermarket shelves are

WHEN THIRST FEELS LIKE HUNGER

Signs of thirst are actually a warning sign that your body is already quite dehydrated and you need to get fluid into you as soon as possible. More often that not, a nagging feeling of hunger, especially if it's not coming up to a mealtime, is actually a dehydration sign. You can get rid of that one easily by drinking glasses of water with your meals, and between them.

pasteurised, a process which gives a longer shelf life but diminishes nutritional value. Also – and all-importantly – sugar as part of the whole fruit has been shown to have less effect on insulin than fruit juice, its extracted form. So for the BTBW Plan, stick to fruit in its natural state.

Smoothies have become so popular over the past few years but, again, moderation is everything as they can be high in sugar. If you enjoy a smoothie, aim to make your own as then you can control what goes into it, and as with the fruit juice, the fresher the better. But do limit your intake to one or two per week.

BOOZE AND THE BTBW PLAN

Next up is alcohol – which in my experience is the single hardest thing to give up people find when they're on a diet. Well the good news is that I am not suggesting that you do give it up, not completely. In moderation, alcohol is a part of life, something many of us enjoy, and that's just fine.

The *type* of alcohol you drink is the most important element when it comes to staying slim and healthy. Beer is certainly out as it is full of yeast, which will give you a big, bloated stomach and can often stay in your stomach for a long time, fermenting, making you even more bloated and gassy. Cider is also out because it is very high in sugar, though some of the organic brands have lesser quantities, so shop around if it's a drink you just can't give up. Wine, both white and red, is ok in moderation – and red wine has antioxidants, which are beneficial to the body, but wine is high in sugar so, again, moderation is everything.

THE BEST BOOZE FOR BTBW

- **Champagne/cava/sparkling wine:** Low in calories and high in bubbles which means that you tend to drink less than you would other drinks.

- **Spirits and mixers:** Spirits are higher in alcohol and low in calories. In terms of mixers, swap high-sugar ones such as Coke or 7-Up with tonic. Avoid the additive-ridden diet alternatives here too. And consider still or sparkling water – they make great mixers too, contain no sugar, and are definitely most BTBW-friendly!

DRINKING CLEVER

Government recommendations for women are not to exceed fourteen units of alcohol over the course of a week. A unit of alcohol is termed a 'standard drink', which is 10g of alcohol. This equates to a small glass of wine (100mls); a glass of lager, cider or stout; or a pub measure of spirit.

When dieting, most people tend to cut out alcohol, which can lead to binge drinking when the diet finishes.

. . . .

Because the BTBW Food Plan is a *way of eating for life* (doesn't that sound better than diet?), we don't recommend you cut out alcohol – but do make sure you drink in moderation. What's set out above is a good rule of thumb.

. . . .

For those special occasions when you may have several drinks in one night, the hangover munchies the next day can be the undoing of a smoothly working BTBW Food Plan. Taking a Dioralyte sachet in water before you go to bed will help with this, cutting down on that craving for white starchy carbohydrates the next day, and helping that dehydration headache. Dioralyte is available from chemists and is simply a mixture of salts, sugars and electrolytes and will stop the body from dehydrating overnight.

EATING OUT THE BTBW WAY

Not only am I telling you that you don't have to give up alcohol, I am also telling you that you don't have to stop eating out in restaurants. Food is such a wonderful part of life and a night out with your friends or partner at a restaurant is a great way to spend time. But you can do a serious amount of damage to your BTBW Food Plan if you choose the wrong options. So below is a simple rule book for eating out:

- Always have a glass of water beside your alcohol glass and switch between the two during the meal.

- Aim to have soup, salad or protein for your starter. If you are ordering a salad, aim to have the dressing on the side and choose the oil-based dressings rather than the creamy, calorie-laden ones.

- Ideally, put your knife and fork down between bites and chew your food.

- For your main meal, have protein and vegetables instead of potatoes or rice, etc, especially if the menu doesn't feature brown carbs, the low GI kind. Vegetables are full of fibre and nutrients so you can load up on them.

- Desserts should be fruit-based or sorbets. If you are going to go for the calorie-laden chocolate cake, then aim for the best one you can get!

EATING FOR WORKING OUT

Many people ask me how they can maximise fat burn during their training sessions. I researched this area as part of my Master's degree and the evidence is that eating only protein and low GI vegetables around two to three hours before your session will gain the best results for you. High GI foods have actually been proven to shut down your body's ability to burn fat.

In terms of post-workout nutrition, you basically have two windows of opportunity to get the nutrients back into your body:

- **20 minutes post session:** This is the time to get some simple carbs back into your body to help replenish your glycogen stores. A piece of fruit is ideal.

- **40 minutes post session:** Here is the time to get the major nutrients back into your body, so it's the time to get a proper meal in, consisting of the major nutrients, protein with plenty of vegetables and some brown carbs will be perfect. So scheduling your mealtimes around your workout sessions, where possible, can have extra beneficial effects.

SUPPLEMENTS

Now more than ever, supplements are increasingly popular. People are attracted by the idea of a magic pill that will change their shape and reduce their weight more quickly and easily, without having to put in the hard work.

Supplements may be trendy, but if weight loss is what you are aiming for, they are never the best way forward. While they may have their place in high-end sports – and endurance athletes often need them to help their bodies recover – they have no place here.

Some supplements claim to force your body to burn fat and in some respects they do, but you can do the same thing by eating more healthily, without the potentially dangerous levels of caffeine and other stimulants that speed up your heart rate and metabolism.

Other supplements claim to reduce fat absorption in your stomach, which may be true, but they will generally lead to gastro-intestinal problems such as diarrhoea, often unexpectedly. I have been giving lectures and seen people suddenly get up and run out of the room to go to the toilet, only to discover later that they were taking these products. Not healthy for your system at all.

Then there is my personal pet hate: the milkshake or powder supplements that act as meal replacements. Replacing healthy, real foods with synthetic, low-calorie powders that contain sweeteners and artificial additives just doesn't make sense for long-term results. And what's the point in putting yourself through all that pain only for the weight to pile back on again as soon as you stop, as your body desperately tries to compensate for what it understands as starvation. You will certainly lose weight quite rapidly, but once you begin to eat real food again, you will find the weight goes back on, very fast! Protein drinks after a workout have become really popular as well, and

THE BTBW FOOD PLAN SAYS:

If something looks too good to be true – promising amazing results without any hard work – then it is. True change can't magically happen with the use of a pill or a tablet. And no pill or tablet can deliver the sense of self-empowerment and achievement that comes from taking your health into your own hands. YOU are the creator of your own future.

these can work if you can't make time for a proper meal, but before you go this route, try to get your protein in real food form first, real food is always better for you than a synthetic version.

TOP TIPS FOR BTBW FOOD PLAN SUCCESS

EAT A DIET FULL OF COLOUR

All of your meals should have plenty of colour, not the artificial type but the natural type! This ensures we get a variety of nutrients into our diet. Vegetables and fruit are packed with fibre, vitamins, minerals and antioxidants and are very low in calories (though as we know, fruit consumption should be limited due to the higher GI values). They help keep you satisfied longer, and are a great snack and can be eaten with every meal.

EAT REGULAR MEALS

Eating meals throughout the day will help keep your metabolism stable as well as burning calories all day long. When you don't eat for an extended amount of time, it actually slows down your body, reducing your natural calorie burning. There is a great debate about three or five meals a day; I tend to use three meals and two snacks. Breakfast is the most important meal, it kick starts your body for the day, so no matter what happens, don't skip it! Your snacks can be fruit or small meals, full of nutrients. No matter what way you choose to eat, make sure you don't overdo sugar and starch levels!

GIVE YOUR STOMACH TIME TO CATCH UP

It takes our bodies ten to fifteen minutes to realise we've had enough to eat. So you need to begin chewing your food and slowing down your eating, and leave your knife and fork down between each chew! Because of this delay in feeling full, it is very easy to eat more than our bodies actually need, leaving us feeling stuffed, with the Christmas Day overfull sensation kicking in, where you are actually made sleep by your body as it needs all your energy to digest the food!

EAT WHOLE FRESH FOODS

In order for processed foods to last so long on our shelves in the supermarkets, they contain preservatives, which in turn deplete the nutrients and vitamins originally found in those foods. When possible, purchase fresh foods and avoid pre-packaged and convenient fast food, as these types of food are typically higher in calories, fat and salt as well as preservatives. If you have local markets in your area, why not pick up your fruit and vegetables there – you will get fresher produce and you will be supporting the local economy too.

GET MOVING

Our bodies were not intended to sit behind a desk all day. We need daily exercise to benefit our overall health and especially to strengthen all our muscles including our heart. Exercise can also help you sleep better and improve your mood, so whether a high-impact workout at the gym or a stroll through the neighbourhood, get moving!

TREAT YOURSELF

We all have those few foods that we know aren't good for us but which we have a hard time avoiding, and the more you tell yourself you can't have them, the more you want them! Eventually you will splurge out and eat as much of that restricted food as you can. So allow yourself a treat from time to time, but remember to keep it within moderation. Once a week you should have a guilt-free treat, this way you aren't cutting the food from your diet, making it a more balanced and effective weight-loss plan. There is actually evidence to support the fact that by having your treat day, your body will lose even more weight as your metabolism speeds up to burn off that food, so it's all good all round!

EAT YOUR WHOLE GRAINS

Whole grains are unrefined products that have maintained their nutrients and fibre content, unlike 'white' products that are processed and have less nutritional value. An additional benefit to eating 100 per cent whole grains, such as breads and pastas, is that they help maintain blood sugar levels with less spiking and crashing throughout the day. Whole grains also keep you fuller for longer.

EAT THE 'RIGHT' FAT

Fat has got a reputation for being bad for us and, in many cases, this is true. But there are healthy fats that our bodies actually need. Overeating saturated fats, such as those found in meat and dairy products, leads to those unwanted pounds as well as increasing your risk of heart disease. Stick to healthy fat sources that are unsaturated, such as olive oil. Good fats are essential for body functions, so don't avoid them!

BEWARE OF LIQUID CALORIES

These types of calories will not fill you up, but they will most certainly add weight. Even the supposedly healthy soft drinks contain huge quantities of sugar – a typical 1.5-litre bottle of flavoured water contains sixteen and a half spoonfuls of sugar!

3

GET READY! THE BTBW FITNESS TEST

'I wasn't under any illusions that I was fit – you know you're not fit if you have to huff and puff running for a bus – but at the same time I was in denial because I didn't want to have to get fit. But I was tired all the time, really low in energy and feeling low in myself too, and the doctor said that introducing exercise would actually help. When I first met Karl and we did the fitness test, I thought I'd be mortified. But he explained with no fuss or fanfare that it's nothing more than a useful indication of where a client is at – so that the best programme for their needs can be created. Instead of being mortified, I was actually motivated – and I never expected just how quickly those results would start to change. I'm fairly fit now – and proud of it. And my energy is way better than before.' – Catherine esting your fitness at the outset is vital to a successful BTBW Plan. In this chapter we'll do some tests that will give you some numbers. These will reflect your fitness as you start out on your BTBW journey. As you progress on it, you will see these numbers improve, and this will give a fantastic boost to your motivation levels, which in turn will push you to work even harder. It's a win-win situation! There are many ways that you can check out your fitness levels, and here I am going to share with you my favourite four methods and reveal exactly what they are testing.

. . . .

The important thing is not where you are now – don't be put off if you discover you are less fit than you thought you were. It's all about finding your baseline, something that you can retest every now and again to see how you are reaping the rewards of your work.

When you begin to see the numbers change, you are seeing the direct results of your lifestyle changes, the improvements that that cardiovascular work is having for your heart and lungs, not to mention your waistline.

. . . .

WEIGHT

There is a myth out there that muscle weighs more than fat – it doesn't. One pound of muscle is the same as one pound of fat – it's the density that differs. Muscle is simply more dense than fat. This means that one pound of muscle takes up less space than the one pound of fat. That 1 pound of muscle also takes more calories just to keep it there. Your body has to work around 10–20 per cent harder just to keep lean muscle tissue on your body. How cool is that!?

A weighing scales is not the be all and end all of losing weight, and we'll talk more about that in a moment. But, as an initial measurement of progress, a weighing scales is really useful. Before you embark on the BTBW Plan, ensure that you have a good set of scales and that it is on a level floor. Don't opt for those scales that record body fat measurement as, in my view, they don't work that well unless you are really spending a lot of money. Aim to weigh yourself once a week on the same day at the same time. You are always heavier in the afternoon – as much as 4 pounds, which is almost 2 kilograms – so chances are you'll feel better if you choose morning time for your weigh.

WEIGHTY FACTS

- 1 stone = 14 pounds or 6.35 kilograms
- Each 1 pound of fat you want to lose contains 3,500 calories, which is roughly twelve chocolate bars.
- During your monthly period, your body retains fluid at a rate of 3–7 pounds for a few days before and after.
- Assuming that weight loss is one of your goals in undertaking the BTBW Plan, you should aim to lose 1.5—2 pounds per week. Losing much more than this generally means that you're losing fluid, especially in the first week as your body is self-regulating, improving its circulation and eliminating toxins.

WHAT IS MY IDEAL WEIGHT?

In my many years working with women on their health and fitness plans, I have come to realise that there is no hard-and-fast rule of thumb for a person's ideal weight. There are methods out there for calculating so-called ideal weight – the most common being Body Mass Index (BMI), Body Fat Measurement and Waist Measurement – but the reality is that we are all different shapes, heights and bone structures and it doesn't work to attempt to classify everyone in the same way.

At the same time, we want some sense of what our ideal weight is, so we can work towards that, right?

Well, yes and no. Numbers are helpful only up to a certain point. Become too fixated on them, and they can become the end in itself. Which is losing sight of the original aim.

Who sets out to lose weight because they want to achieve a number?

. . . .

In my experience, women want to lose weight because they're tired of not being able to wear the clothes they like wearing.

Or run for the bus. They want to feel energetic like they used to. Or feel sexy about themselves. They are concerned for their health. There are lots of reasons, and combinations of reasons, and none of them have to do with numbers. Which is why the BTBW Plan has developed other ways of measuring progress.

. . . .

THE SHAKE TEST

So, how do you decide on your ideal weight without relying on the scales? Here's what I recommend – it may not be scientific, but it will give a good indication! Stand in front of a full-length mirror fully naked. Shake yourself about. See what moves. This is your body fat. As you progress on your BTBW Plan, try this once a week, and watch the difference all your hard work is making, as your body fat lowers. Regardless of age, you will see a difference – as your diet gives you back your waist, and the exercises improve your tone.

When the shake test no longer has much shake in it, chances are you're close to if not at your ideal weight.

MEASUREMENTS

However, it can be very satisfying in the early stages of a weight-loss plan to be able to measure progress in inches/cms, as it reinforces the rewards of our hard work. This is why I recommend buying a tape measure. Seeing the numbers below change will help you to stay motivated. Here is a simple table that you can fill in to track your progress.

	Start	Week 1	Week 2	Week 3	Week 4
Weight (in lbs or kilos)					
Neck (in inches or cms)					
Right arm (widest point)					
Bust/Back (nipple line)					
Waist (belly button)					
Hips (widest point)					
Right leg (halfway point)					
Right calf (widest point)					

RESTING HEART RATE

You have measured your weight and your inches, and now you want to see how fit your heart/lungs are. This is something you can find out simply by taking your resting heart rate. This is really easy. Place your right index finger and middle finger roughly an inch under the right side of your jaw. You should feel your pulse almost instantly. You can also use the wrist method, placing your left index and middle finger at the base of your wrist. This can be slightly harder to detect but between these two tests you will be able to find your pulse. This is best done first thing in the morning before you get out of bed. Simply take your pulse for fifteen seconds and multiply the rate by four. The lower the number, the fitter you are.

. . . .

Resting heart rate

Above seventy: need to get fit

Below seventy: reasonable fitness

Below sixty: fit

Below fifty: very fit

Below forty: you must be running marathons!

Once you see your resting heart rate beginning to drop down, you can see that your fitness levels are improving, and high five to that!

. . . .

If your number is over seventy, you really need to get exercising, gently and slowly, but you will be seeing big improvements very quickly.

BODY FITNESS

There are two tests that I am going to show you to measure your body's fitness levels. They are simple to do and will give you an accurate, quick gauge of how fit you are. All you will need is a clock, it's that simple!

. . . .

Ideally do both body fitness tests in the same session. Take a four-minute break between each test to allow your heart rate to settle back down to a normal level.

. . . .

Test 1: Abdominal strength

You will see and hear the word 'core' used all the time in fitness magazines and around gyms, etc. It refers to the area between your bust and your pelvis, all the way around your body. Your posture, back health and flat stomach all depend on you having a strong core. Below is an easy and quick way to test yours.

- Lie on your back on the floor with your knees bent

- Place your hands on your thighs and start to sit up, keeping your eyes looking towards the ceiling so as not to strain your neck

- As you sit up, squeeze your stomach, and come up high enough for your hands to touch your knees

- NB: Keep your head totally relaxed.

I see people all the time who use their hands to drag their neck, but all you're doing here is damaging your neck, I'm afraid. If you get any neck pain at all, be sure to stop straight away. Do as many sit-ups as you can in one minute and compare with the chart below for your results.

Age	18–25	26–35	36–45	46–55	56–65	65+
Excellent	>43	>39	>33	>27	>24	>23
Good	37–43	33–39	27–33	22–27	18–24	17–23
Above average	33–36	29–32	23–26	18–21	13–17	14–16
Average	29–32	25–28	19–22	14–17	10–12	11–13
Below average	25–28	21–24	15–18	10–13	7–9	5–10
Poor	18–24	13–20	7–14	5–9	3–6	2–4
Very poor	<18	<20	<7	<5	<3	<2
My score:						

Test 2: Upper body strength

For this test, we use the age-old press-up test. Here we'll do the easier version of the press-up.

- Go on all fours, knees shoulder-width apart, hips at a 45-degree angle to the floor, and a nice straight back

- Bend your elbows, bringing your chest to the floor and straight back up

- In one minute, do as many as you can until there is no more strength in your arms. Then check your progress with the chart below.

Age	17–19	20–29	30–39	40–49	50–59	60–65
Excellent	>35	>36	>37	>31	>25	>23
Good	27–35	30–36	30–37	25–31	21–25	19–23
Above average	21–27	23–29	22–30	18–24	15–20	13–18
Average	11–20	12–22	10–21	8–17	7–14	5–12
Below average	6–10	7–11	5–9	4–7	3–6	2–4
Poor	2–5	2–6	1–4	1–3	1–2	1
Very poor	0–1	0 1	0	0	0	0
My score:						

These tests will give you a great idea of how fit or unfit you are. Regardless of the results, this is *your* starting point. We all need one, it provides a great way for you to measure your progress. Retest yourself after four weeks and you will be amazed at the changes. You don't have to use both the tests, simply take the one that suits you best and follow that one.

4

BURN THOSE CALORIES! THE BTBW CARDIO PLAN

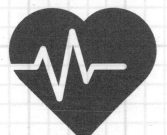

'Running has given me all that I thought it would and so much more. It gives me time to process the day, solve the problems, come up with answers and make plans. Every run, love it or hate it, blows off the cobwebs, gives a sense of achievement and brings renewed energy for the next one.' – Gemma

Cardiovascular work is a key part of any training plan, and an element that you simply can't do without. It constitutes anything that gets your heart rate up and your lungs working, forcing your body to burn carbohydrates, then fat, as its primary fuel source. If you exercise at the right level, you can increase the amount of fat that your body burns. That's right, burning fat as the main fuel source, this is what you should be aiming for.

THE TALK TEST

The best way to know if you're doing this is the talk test.

. . . .

You should always be able to talk while walking, cycling or running, but be somewhat out of breath. If you can't talk at all, you are working too hard! However, the opposite is the most common mistake people make when exercising, they don't work hard enough to get the maximum benefit from their session. You should be able to talk, but not too much!

. . . .

A stroll of a walk is good to loosen your body out, but does little good for the layer of wine wobble around your waistline; you need to push yourself that little bit harder to properly reap the benefits. Get that heart rate up, but not too much, to ensure that you are burning the fuel that you want to be. Your breathing should be elevated, but not overly so. Combining a proper cardiovascular workout with resistance training – a fancy term for exercises – gives you the most powerful tool you will ever need to get your body in shape quickly and effectively! Combine these with a kick-ass food plan like the one I have given you, and you have everything you will ever need to get the results you have always wanted.

WHAT IS CARDIOVASCULAR WORK?

Literally, anything that gets your pulse up and lungs working, for example:

- Brisk walking

- Running

- Swimming

- Cycling

- Surfing

- Sex!

These are some prime examples, but it can be any sport that you enjoy – because the more you enjoy it, the longer you will keep it up. Who cares what the latest fad workout is at the moment if you absolutely hate doing it, because it will just be a short-term attempt at getting fit. Keep trying as many sports as you can until you find one that you enjoy!

THE IMPORTANCE OF CARDIO IN THE BTBW PLAN

Think of that chocolate bar you had last night. Those squares that tasted so, so good. A brisk one-hour walk will help to burn off those calories – all 300 of them. Resistance workouts – the BTBW Exercise Plan – will burn lots of calories as well and help kick start your metabolism, but cardiovascular sessions are crucial to any fitness plan.

. . . .

The BTBW 1/3 Rule:
1 HOUR OF CARDIO EXERCISE, 3 TIMES A WEEK.
Break it into 30-minute segments if time necessitates, but however you achieve it, never forget the 1/3 Rule.

. . . .

DO I HAVE TO RUN FOR MY BTBW PLAN?

There is a big trend for running at the moment, and personally I think it is one of the best forms of cardio exercise and a wonderful tool in the BTBW Plan. When I first broach the topic of running with my clients, they often say that they can't run, or don't like running. If you're not fit, then I would expect that you don't like running – it makes you out of breath and tired, you have to stop before you have a chance to reap all the wonderful benefits of endorphin (happy hormone) release, and the whole experience just reinforces the unpleasant truth that you are unfit!

But the BTBW Running Plan will show you how to run at your level, and not get out of breath, and I advise that you give it a chance before you decide that running is not for you.

 The other side of this, though, is that running isn't for everyone, and if you've given it a chance and you find it's really not for you, you don't need to worry! There are plenty of other options, equally good.

TWO-SPEED SETTING: THE FAT-BURNING SECRET WEAPON

Whatever your level of fitness, and whatever your sport, 'intervals' are the secret key to getting your body fat down and knocking inches off your body. Intervals mean exercising using two speeds – just like the gears of a car. And they are really easy to do.

No matter what your sport, you can apply them. Your first speed setting is slow and steady, the second is fast. You design your plan with these in mind, initially a large steady interval and a small fast interval such as:

FIVE MINUTES SLOW, TWO MINUTES FAST.

As you get fitter, you begin to lower the slow interval and increase the fast interval:

THREE MINUTES SLOW AND FOUR MINUTES FAST.

And when you get really fit you can lower the easy interval again:

ONE MINUTE SLOW AND SIX MINUTES FAST.

Following are four cardio plans: Walking, Running,

BTBW INTERVAL RULE OF THUMB

All you need to ensure is that you are working as hard as you can on the fast interval and going easy and steady on the slow interval. The function of the slow interval is simply to let your body recover and bring your heart rate back down before you attack the next fast one. It is also the best time to take some water on board as you psyche yourself up and knuckle down for the next one.

Cycling and Swimming. First decide which one is for you, then simply follow the steps provided.

BIG STEPS: THE BTBW WALKING PLAN

Walking is one of the cheapest, easiest and most effective ways to get fit, lose weight and get healthy. To get started, I advise that you get gait analysis, to ensure that you have the correct runners for your foot type. This is offered free in most sports stores around the country. It simply ensures that your feet are properly supported, keeping your joints safe and reducing the chances of getting those annoying blisters.

. . . .

Remember your BTBW 1/3 Rule: you should be aiming for a one-hour brisk walk, three times a week. Done right, this is sufficient to get results. The important part of any walk is your speed. You need to be covering 4 miles (or 6.4 kilometres) per hour to get the maximum benefits. Sound fast? Well it is. No strolling or stopping to chat to neighbours, this is your time to push your body.

. . . .

Remember, the four-mile walk is your aim – depending on your fitness level, it may not be possible starting off. IN THIS CASE, START WITH THIRTY MINUTES AND BUILD UP TO THE MAGIC HOUR OVER THE COURSE OF TWO OR THREE WEEKS. Set this as one of your goals. For some people, walking for fifteen minutes a day is a huge challenge, but use this to your advantage and set your goals to build it up, adding up to five minutes every day. Reward yourself and keep working at it.

Below is a chart to help figure what you should be aiming for. This is your guide – if you can exceed its expectations, then by all means, do!

To measure your walking route

- Drive it in your car and record the distance

- Use an online mapping route such as www.mapmyrun.com or aaroutefinder

- Use a mobile phone app such as runkeeper or mapmyrun

- Use a GPS watch, such as those by Garmin.

By measuring the distance, you can ensure that you are working hard enough, and once you hit the magic four miles per hour, aim to do it even faster using the goal-setting techniques we discussed earlier in the book.

What else should you look out for to improve your walking workout once you get fit?

- **Change your route weekly.** Your body regularly needs new challenges to maximise the effect of exercise, so add in some hills or even reverse your current route

- **Change your stride.** Shorten or lengthen your stride during the walk to ensure you are mixing up the muscle groups that are being worked

- **Change your speed.** As we looked at effective before, constantly trying to improve your speed is the simplest and often most way of increasing the difficulty of your walk. Use intervals to push yourself.

. . . .

YOUR FOUR-WEEK WALKING AIM
Beginners: At the end of the four weeks you should be aiming to walk four miles in under an hour.
Moderate: Make sure you keep changing your routes to get the maximum benefit

from your fast walks. Use the talk test to ensure you are working hard enough.

Advanced: After four weeks, you should be setting personal best times for your four-mile walks and starting into a little running.

. . . .

RUN FREE: THE BTBW RUNNING PLAN

I've spoken of my enthusiasm for running. As I tell all my clients, anyone can run, regardless of your level of fitness. And, with a little bit of hard work and some guidance, running is something that you can grow to enjoy. It has fast become one of the most popular sports on the planet, with races of different distances happening almost every weekend throughout the year. Running is not primarily about losing weight, it is about the joy of feeling fit, of watching the world go by using your feet to propel you.

Start your run like this:

Get on your shoes and out you go. For the first

EASY OFF THE BLOCKS

No doubt some of you will have tried to run before, and failed to keep it up. And I would bet that you made one key mistake, however unintentional. Often when we start off a new form of exercise, in our initial burst of enthusiasm we start off too fast. By doing this, our heart rate increases rapidly and our lungs can't catch up, and we get that awful panic breathing that causes so much discomfort and forces you to stop. Sound familiar? I am going to show you a different way, an easier way, a way that will get you running safely and efficiently.

two minutes, focus on your breathing, in through your nose and out through your mouth. Keep your mind focused on this and you will soon notice it start to settle.

. . . .

Let your breathing, rather than your pace, be your guide.

. . . .

If you've experienced that breathing discomfort in the past, you'll feel the difference now. This is because you are easing your body into the run, slowly but surely, and allowing yourself time to adjust.

Keep it up for as long as you can, recording the number of minutes. Use this number as the base of your training plan.

Aim to run three times per week, using your recorded number of minutes as your fast interval, and introducing a slow one in between in the form of a brisk walk, to allow you time to recover. For example, if your fast interval is ten minutes, make your slow interval two minutes, and repeat five times. This gives you a one-hour session with plenty of recovery time. Over the course of four weeks, you simply increase your fast interval and reduce your slow one.

If, in time, you want to train for a 5-kilometre or 10-kilometre race, then you can use the training plans at the back of the book.

. . . .

YOUR FOUR-WEEK RUNNING AIM

Beginners: After four weeks you should be able to run consistently for up to 20 minutes.

Moderate: After four weeks you should be able to run 5k, so why not register for a 5k race?

Advanced: Aim to increase your speed over the four weeks by using interval training and register for races to see what your personal best is.

. . . .

ON YOUR BIKE! THE BTBW CYCLING PLAN

Another one of the booming sports in the past few years has been cycling. Providing a serious workout without the joint impact of running, cycling is an ideal way to see the world and get fit at the same time. You can burn up to 800 calories per hour on a bike, working your bum, legs, waist and, surprisingly, arms all at the same time. And it's easy to get into: all you need is a bike and a helmet and off you go.

If you don't already have a bike, and are considering buying one, for the BTBW Plan I recommend a hybrid type: it has the comfort of a mountain bike and the speed of a racer. They are great on the flats and going up hills, around town and generally easy to use anywhere. If you're planning on cycling routes that are very hilly, a racer is worth considering, as they are fast, light and have really thin tyres. However, they're less comfortable than a hybrid and also prone to slippiness in wet weather.

If you find you enjoy cycling and want to do more, it's worth investing in a decent pair of Lycra-padded shorts. Yes, they can be somewhat embarrassing, but they are seriously comfortable and will stop you from getting the sore bum that comes from spending time in the saddle. Another accessory that will make life easier but can take some getting used to is some cleats. Cleats are the cycling shoes that clip you into the bike, giving you more power in your push. But be careful, and make sure you are confident in using them before you set out, otherwise you run the risk of a fall!

When figuring out your cycling plan, remember the BTBW 1/3 Rule – aim to be cycling one hour three times a week. Choose a round route that includes a variety of terrain – flat only is not going to get the heart pumping as you need it.

If you are taking up cycling for the first time or haven't been on a bike for a long time, try this 4-week plan to see rapid benefits:

- **Week 1:** Spend this week finding your balance, comfort and steadiness on your bike, get used to the gears, saddle and pedal stroke

- **Week 2:** Now you have the basics, cycle some routes that you enjoy and time yourself, being careful not to push too hard

- **Week 3:** Now you can push a little harder on the bike, improving your times and your technique as you become more and more comfortable with the bike

- **Week 4:** Why not add in some intervals, pushing a hard gear for two minutes and an easy gear for two minutes, this will help develop leg power and challenge the muscles more.

. . . .

YOUR FOUR-WEEK CYCLING AIM

Beginners: Use the first few weeks to get used to cycling, gaining confidence on the road, by week four starting on intervals.

Moderate: Use the four weeks to increase your distance and speed so that your body is always challenged.

Advanced: Why not time yourself over a certain distance in week one and then try again three weeks later. Watch the benefits of all your hard work.

. . . .

TAKE THE PLUNGE: THE BTBW SWIMMING PLAN

Swimming is a wonderful form of cardiovascular exercise and is less hard on the body than running. But beware: gently swimming up and down the pool for twenty minutes won't burn many calories, or stress your muscles to the extent that you will see a difference. While it will loosen up your joints and is a good way to relax, here we are looking for a different kind of result. You need to knuckle down and push your body a little harder to get a really good workout!*

Here's how to maximise that session, the BTBW way:

- **Mix it up:** A mix of the three main strokes – front crawl, breaststroke and backstroke – is most effective and will deliver a great session once you are working hard enough.

- **Plan the session:** Regardless of what stroke you are using, the structure of the

---

*The BTBW Swimming Plan assumes that you know the basic strokes involved: the front crawl, breaststroke and backstroke. If you don't, you will need to learn these because otherwise you won't be able to get the type of cardio workout you need. Check out your local swimming pool or gym for lessons.

session is all-important to your workout. A gentle session might burn 150 calories in 30 minutes, but a tough session can burn up to 500. There is that much of a difference, that's basically one large chocolate bar you are burning! Your session should consist of one or two gentle lengths to warm up your body and get the blood flowing ready for your session. This helps your body to loosen out and helps prevent injury too. Then comes the main body of the session – which you will be working towards at the outset: AT LEAST 1,000 METRES (40 LENGHTS IN A 25M POOL) OF HARD WORK.

- **Use intervals:** These are essential to getting you the results you want, as opposed to just swimming up and down the pool for the whole session. Not only does this get monotonous, but you're not making the most of your time! The interval could be made up of any different combination of lengths, e.g. 50 metres fast, 50 slow to begin with; as fitness improves, 100 metres fast,

50 metres slow; moving towards 200 metres fast, 50 metres slow. And so forth.

- **Adapt your session:** Remember, your results simply plateau if your body isn't challenged enough, so ideally you should be adapting your sessions as much as possible. As you increase your fast and reduce your slow intervals, this will ensure that you are constantly pushing your body a little harder each time, which means that your workout is always tough enough to produce results and get you the results you want.

FANCY AN EASY SWIMMING SESSION?
If you have done a weights session or tough run, an easy swim is a good way to ease your muscles out, leaving you fresh and ready for your next session. Enjoy!

- **Remember your BTBW 1/3 Rule:** three one-hour sessions per week.

. . . .

YOUR FOUR-WEEK SWIMMING AIM

Beginners: Swimming can be quite scary, so the first four weeks may just be getting comfortable in the water, realising just how good it feels to be swimming.

Moderate: Once you are comfortable in the water you should be aiming to work harder during your swim sessions, improving your speed and technique.

Advanced: Test your 100m personal best and try to improve it each week, especially in week four!

. . . .

5

ROCK THAT SHAPE: THE BTBW EXERCISES!

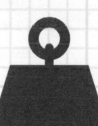

'I'm not going to pretend I relish an exercise workout – especially not just before it! But I'll say this much for nothing – I relish the shape it's given me. And to be honest, I don't really think twice about doing the BTBW exercises anymore, they've become like second nature. And, with the radio in the background and no one there to disturb me, I'm happy out.' – Mary

Now that we have a new, healthier diet on stream and a cardiovascular plan in place, we can start to look at the all-important exercises that are going to transform your bum, tum and bingo wings to create the toned look you desire.

In the following sections you will see three levels of workout. Start with level one and progress to level two after two weeks (or sooner depending on your fitness). Once the workouts at level two become manageable, you can progress to level three. There are two exercises in each level, and to achieve the results you want, you will need to do these three times a week.

REPS AND SETS

These refer to the number of times you repeat an exercise.

Reps is short for repetitions and simply stands

for the number of times you repeat an exercise movement.

A set occurs when you have completed the required number of reps.

. . . .

BTBW SETS/REPS RULE OF THUMB
20 reps per exercise = 1 set
10–15 second break between sets
Complete 3 sets

. . . .

You know by now how fit you are, and how much you need to improve. To help you understand how best to approach the exercises, we'll use three categories; you'll know to which one you belong:

- **Beginners:** Anyone who is just starting on the road to fitness. You should take it easy when starting this plan. Initially start with one set and gradually build up to two and three sets over the course of time. Ensure to drink plenty of water and exercise in a well-ventilated room, taking breaks when you need to.

- **Moderate:** If you have a good level of fitness to start with, then you can push yourself harder with this plan. You will progress quickly to level two and three of the exercises and can push yourself harder as you will have a greater base level of fitness.

- **Advanced:** Those of you who are already fit can start at level two and progress to level three very quickly. You may already have an exercise plan so you can add some of these exercises in to achieve even better results than those you are already getting.

It is important to take a break whenever you feel the need to. If you feel that you are pushing your body too hard or feel sick/dizzy or nauseous, then stop straight away. These are extreme symptoms, and you should be taking enough breaks so that you don't get to the point of feeling unwell. When you need to, drink water between sets. Ensure that the room you are exercising in is well ventilated with plenty of fresh air as these are two major factors that will have a big influence on your workout.

DON'T FORGET TO BREATHE

Many people forget to breathe properly when they work out, and so make their bodies work a lot harder than they need to. By breathing properly, you are getting essential oxygen into your muscles and getting rid of carbon dioxide. Aim to breathe in on the easy part of the exercise and breathe out on the hard part, it is that simple. The better you breathe, the more benefits you will get from your sessions and the better you will feel!

BUILDING IT UP

Begin at the first level and gradually build your way up steadily. If you jump in feet first and do the advanced ones straight away, you run the risk of serious muscle fatigue, which can not only make simple tasks, such as drying your hair, painful, but is also a great de-motivator. When you build up fitness slowly, not only do you gain confidence in your ability, you gain motivation.

. . . .

Remember, this book is a long-term plan,
not a quick fix – it's not only acceptable,
it's actually best practice to build up the
routines over a number of weeks and keep
in mind that the results are exponential
– that is the great thing. As you build up
your fitness level, you come to reap more
and more from each session.

. . . .

It is all about achieving measurable results, but
it's a continuous plan – my goal for you is to be
exercising a year from now, and for it to be such
an integral part of your regular routine that it's no
longer a drag, but something you look forward to.
And believe me, it is achievable, because exercise
becomes a healthy addiction. All those endorphins
being released means that you get such a buzz from
it that it becomes pay-off in itself. Prepare to reap
the benefits!

GOOD PAIN AND BAD PAIN – THE DIFFERENCE

The old adage 'no pain, no gain' is true to an extent. But there is a remarkable difference between sore muscle pain from exercise and serious pain that indicates a tear or strain. You need to ensure that you do the exercises gradually to reduce the chance of injury. When during exercise you feel some pain coming into your muscles, continue to work out as long as you can keep the technique correct. As soon as your technique begins to suffer, stop straight away.

By ensuring you are doing the exercises correctly, you will stay safe and exercise for longer. Pain that indicates muscle damage tends to be shorter and sharper and more intense – if you feel this, then you should immediately stop and implement the RICE principles set out below, as you would to manage any injury:

- **Rest:** Stop what you are doing and immediately rest your body to prevent inflicting any further damage to the affected area.

118

- **Ice:** Apply ice or a pack of frozen vegetables to the area of pain as this will help to reduce the swelling and bruising. Check the area every two minutes to see if there is redness around the skin, as this is an indicator of ice burn – if you see it, stop straight away. If the ice is too cold, you can wrap a towel around it and this will make it far more useable.

- **Compression:** Applying pressure to the area using a strap or some compression clothing will reduce the swelling and improve your recovery time. Ensure that the pressure isn't too tight and isn't stopping proper circulation to the area.

- **Elevation:** By elevating the area, you are reducing the swelling and improving your recovery time. Use a pillow or a chair for lower body injuries.

Let us begin the BTBW Exercise Plan!

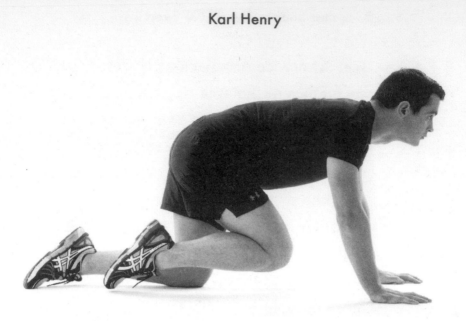

BUMS

Ok, now that you're fully in the picture, it's time to get down to work. Prepare to be introduced to your exercise plan to lift, tone and firm up that bum.

LEVEL ONE

- **Bum kicks:** *A bum-toning classic.*

  - Kneel on the floor on all fours and ensure your back is flat

  - Bring your right knee into your chest and kick the right leg back away from you, so that it is aligned with your back

- Ensure you squeeze your bum as you push your leg out

- Repeat 20 times in and out. Hold for 20 seconds

- Repeat on left leg

- Take a ten-second break before moving on to your second set

- Repeat three sets.

NOTE: If your back gets sore, go down onto your elbows as this will add extra support for your body.

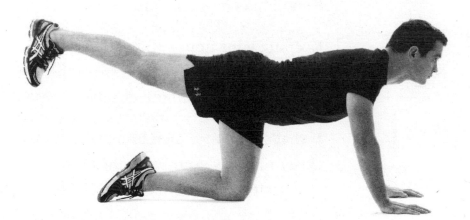

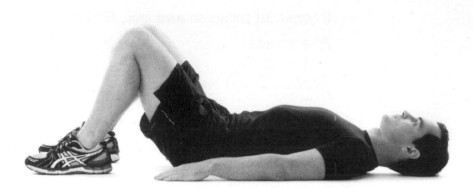

- **Pelvic floor kicks:** *Simple to do and extremely effective.*

  - Lie on your back on the floor, knees bent, hands by your side

  - Keeping your upper body relaxed, simply push your pelvis towards the ceiling, using your bum cheeks

  - If that's too easy, then bring your feet closer towards your bum; the closer in your feet are, the harder it will get. If you have any back pain, then push your feet a little farther away from your bum. The more you squeeze your bum, the greater the effect

- Complete 20 reps for each set. The first set may seem very easy but as you progress to the second and third sets, this exercise gets that little bit harder.

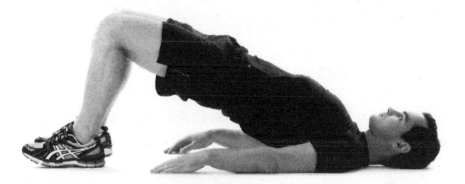

Now that you have mastered the first two exercises, it is time to make things a little more challenging for you. Keep up the good work and remember to ensure that your technique is correct.

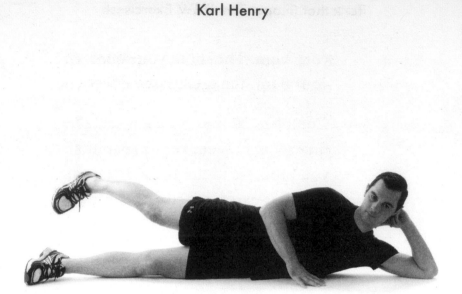

LEVEL TWO

- **Rear-side leg raises:** *An adaptation of the classic side leg raise.*

  - Lie on your left or right side, joints – shoulders, hips, knees and ankles – aligned

  - Keeping your top leg straight, move it behind your body. This engages the bum and forces it to work

- Keep your leg behind your body and raise it up and down as much as your flexibility will allow

- Do 20 reps on your right side and then repeat on your left side = 1 set

- Take a short break between sets, complete three.

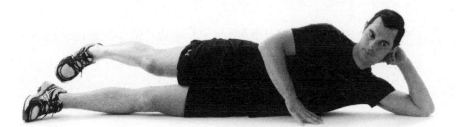

- **Knee in, leg out:** *This exercise is great when it is combined with the rear-side leg raise.*

  - Lie on your left or right side, joints aligned

  - Bring the knee of your top leg in towards your chest and then push it away from your body. Squeeze your bum on the way out

  - Complete your twenty reps on the first side, switch sides and repeat

  - Do three sets.

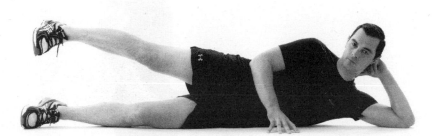

Now it's time to make things a little harder again. The next level will push the body a little more – aim for these once you have completed levels one and two.

LEVEL THREE

- **Step-ups:** *Work your aerobic system, bum, quads and hamstrings. A complete lower body exercise. Very effective in lifting and toning your bum.*

    - Start with a step, bench or chair – the

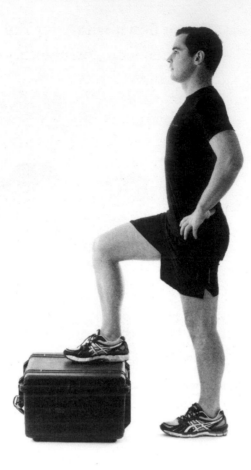

minimum height is ten inches (25 centimetres) but you can go higher as you get fitter. Stand facing it

- Keep your posture straight and tall. Put your hands on your hips. Step up with your right leg, then step up with your left leg

- T step down with your right leg and then step down with your left leg

- This counts as one rep

- Continue leading with the right leg for twenty reps and then lead with

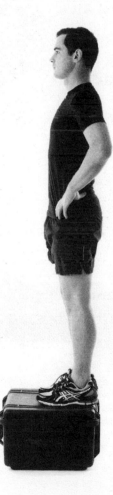

your left leg for 20 reps. This counts as one set

- Take a break, take some water when you need to and then start into your second and third sets.

- **Angled bum kicks:** *One of the best for toning the bum muscles.*

  - Go on all fours

  - Kick out your right leg so that it is parallel to the floor

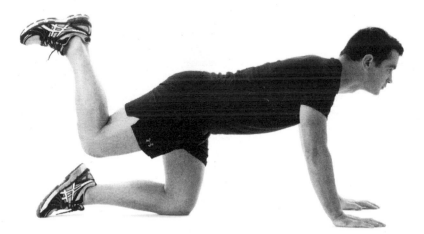

- Bend at the knee

- Push right foot up towards the ceiling

- Repeat whole for 20 reps and then bring your right leg back to all fours

- Switch to your left leg and repeat for twenty reps. This counts as one set

- Complete three sets.

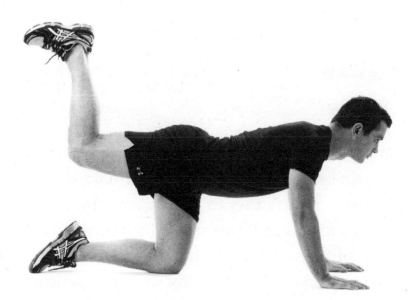

THE ORANGE-PEEL EFFECT

If we are carrying excess weight, chances are we know all about the orange-peel effect beneath our skin: cellulite. This is ordinary body fat sitting under the skin in tiny pockets separated by connective tissue. The most enjoyable way to rid yourself of the dreaded cellulite is some deep tissue massage. Ideally the best way to get this done is by a good, strong and firm masseuse, but you can get your partner to work on your legs, using a rolling pin, literally rolling the affected skin (though put some oils on the skin first to take some of the pain away). You can scream your heart out as the rolling pin helps to get the fat moving. Combine this with plenty of water in your diet, add a little lemon, and you will help to flush the released fat out of your system.

TUMS

When I first assess what a new client is looking for, it's almost inevitable that a flat tummy is top of the list – and it's easy to understand why. A toned tummy looks good, your clothes feel better to wear, and, all importantly, a flat tummy means you've lost that bloated feeling that many women experience.

THE HIDDEN SIX-PACK

Despite what you might think, the biggest key to a flat tummy is food. Only after your diet is working right do you get the full benefit of a tummy-toning workout.

. . . .

You might be surprised to know that you already have a six-pack. We all do. The difference between us all is what covers that six-pack. And while doing sit-ups will help tone your muscles, it won't affect the fat surrounding them in the least. I get tired reading articles recommending hundreds of sit-ups as the key to a flatter tum when the reality is that your diet is the most important part initially.

. . . .

The BTBW Food Plan is exactly what I recommend to my own clients, and all the evidence shows that it works. Low GI foods are low in the substances, such as starch and yeast, that cause bloating. White carbs are the worst offenders when it comes to bloating, followed a close second by beer and cider.

But, of course, to maximise that flatter tummy that will come from our food plan, you're looking for better tone, and this comes from exercise. These exercises, used as part of your overall plan, will create the tone you desire. And they're not just for the centre of your tummy either; all-importantly, they will work the sides of your body and the lower part too – the whole tummy area. There are no Swiss balls needed for this section as you simply don't need them to get results. Also, using Swiss balls without a personal trainer or fitness instructor beside you can actually be dangerous as they are so unstable. By keeping the exercises simple yet effective, I know that you are doing them correctly at home.

So, let's take a look.

LEVEL ONE

- **Pullover:** *A great exercise to stretch out your arms, shoulders, back, chest and stomach area. Note: Try different weights to get one that gives you the best full stretch.*

    - Get two 500ml bottles of water or light dumbbells

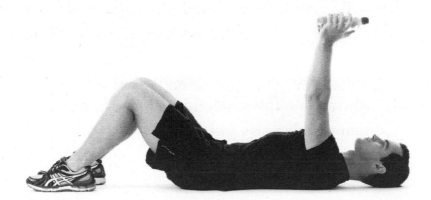

- Lie on the floor with your knees bent

- Hold the dumbbells above your belly button with your arms straight. Keeping your arms straight, lower the bottles back towards the floor

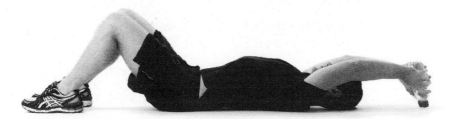

- Do 20 reps, three sets.

· ·

This exercise also works great at the end of your session as it helps to stretch out so many body parts, helping to avoid muscle pain the following day!

· ·

- **Hands to knees sit-ups:** *A great one to work the stomach a little harder.*

  - Lie on your back, knees bent. (By having your knees bent, you are forcing the lower back into the floor, keeping it safe)

- Place your hands on your legs and relax your neck

- Keep your chin up and your neck relaxed and look up at the ceiling throughout

- As you raise your body up, no more than three or four inches, move your hands up your legs towards your knees

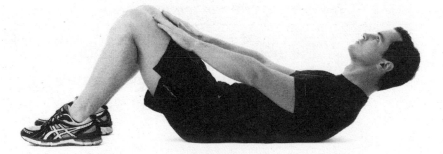

- Return to the floor

- Do 20 reps, three sets.

· ·

If you do this exercise properly, there's no reason for you to strain your neck (eyes to the ceiling) or back (pressed into the floor). If you do experience discomfort, check yourself, only raise yourself up to the point of no neck or back pain, and progress from there. As your core strength builds, any discomfort will decrease.

· ·

LEVEL TWO

- **Bridge:** *A classic stomach/back exercise, extremely effective in toning the tum.*

  - Lie on your front, elbows on the floor, shoulder-width apart, hands pointing away from you

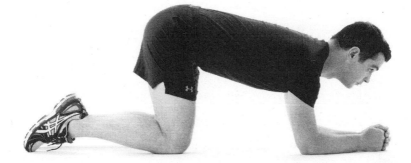

- Point your feet so that you're resting on your toes

- Keeping your back and legs straight, raise your body off the ground.

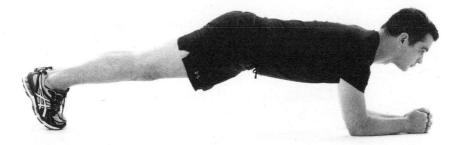

Hold in this position for up to thirty
seconds, or as long as you can,
pulling your belly button towards
your spine, ensuring that your back is
totally flat

- Repeat three times.

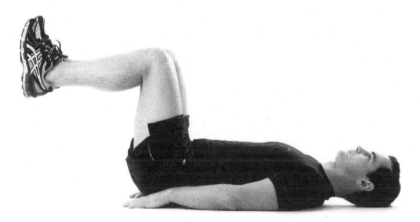

- **Pilates sit-up:** *Involves very little
movement but don't be fooled!*

  - Lie on the floor, back pushed into it

  - Bend knees to 45 degrees (feet off the

floor so that your shins are parallel with it)

- Hold for 30 seconds

- Extend right leg out as far as feels comfortable. The lower you extend the leg, the more your back is forced to work, so be careful

- Return to 45-degree bend

- Extend left leg

- Repeat three times.

As with all the exercises, stop if you feel pain.

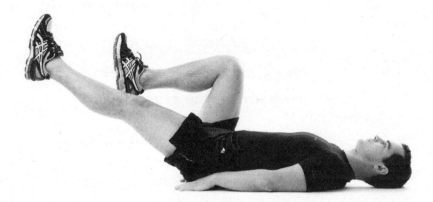

LEVEL THREE

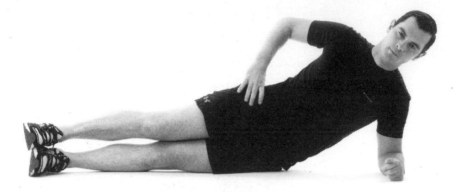

- **Side bridge:** *Excellent for the side waist (oblique and intercostal) muscles.*

  - Lie on your right side, joints aligned

  - Resting on right elbow (using left arm for balance if needs be) raise your body off the ground

  - Make sure legs and back are straight

  - Hold for thirty seconds, ensuring that

your right elbow is directly under your right shoulder

- Switch sides, repeat on left side

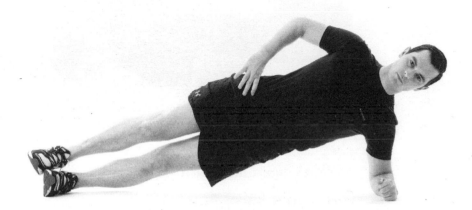

- Repeat three times.

• **Knees in/legs out:** *A great way to hit the lower abdominal and pelvic muscles.*

- Lie on your back, hands under bum

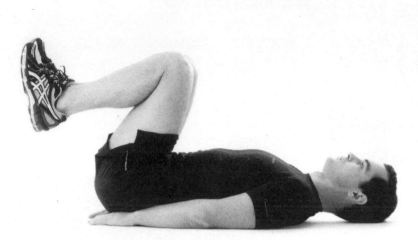

- With head and shoulders on floor, lift your knees and bring them in towards your chest

- Extend legs away from your body, as far as you feel comfortable (the farther and lower they are kicked away, the harder and more effective it will be)

- Do 20 reps, three sets.

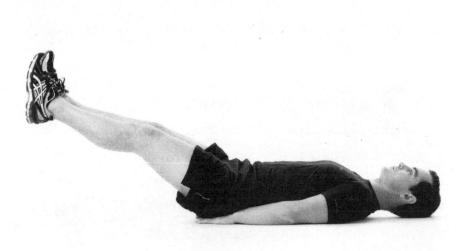

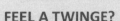

FEEL A TWINGE?

With stomach exercises, you need to be very careful of your lower back, especially when starting out, because the weaker the core, the harder it has to work. At the slightest twinge in your lower back, you should stop straight away. I work with so many people who have back problems, and taking due precaution, we work to build up their strength over time, slowly and safely. As the back strengthens, inevitably the back problems reduce.

BINGO WINGS

If you're familiar with the term bingo wings, then chances are there's a reason. When we are carrying excess weight, it's very natural for the soft tissue at the back of our arms to become affected, creating the flabbiness that women become most aware of when the weather gets warmer and the time comes to expose the arms.

As I mention in the Introduction, the triceps are the muscle group responsible, and this part of the body can deteriorate quickly, from your mid-twenties onwards – although increasingly I am seeing cases in younger people too. I believe that diet plays a significant role in this, and a diet that is high in white carbs and heavy in processed foods is a big factor.

As we age, fat gets stored in several places and the back of the arm is one of them, particularly in women. There is a commonly held myth that this happens when muscle gets turned into fat but this is, in fact, a scientific impossibility. What actually happens is that as we age, our bodies naturally reduce the amount of lean muscle tissue we have and increase the amount of fat stores. This natural process, when combined with a lack of resistance exercise and a poor diet, is a recipe for disaster, and you end up with soft, flabby arms that you do not want to reveal.

. . . .

The good news is that, using the exercises I'm about to outline, combined with your new diet, you can firm up, tone up and shape up your arms no matter what shape they are in. I have seen incredible results over the years with clients who have gained definition in their arms and changed their whole wardrobe around the fact that they wanted to show them off.

. . . .

In my eyes, a toned, shapely arm is the best look for women, I think that the thicker look should be left for the men – call me old school but that is what I think looks best and that is the look that I am aiming to give you.

THE BARE ARM TEST

Stand in front of the mirror in your bra or vest top and take a minute to look at your arms. Raise one arm in the air and give it a shake – is there too much loose skin moving around for your liking? Would you like to improve it? If the answer is yes, take a mental note of that feeling, because the will to change is one serious motivation. If you follow my advice, you will see a discernible difference in the shape of your arms in just a few weeks. It will take hard work, but the end result will make it all worthwhile – when you slip into that dress and have arms to be proud of, that you will want to show off again.

So, here are the exercises to add into your routine.

LEVEL ONE

- **Triceps dips:** *The classic triceps exercise. Can be done at home or even when you are out on your walk.*

  - Sit on the edge of a bench or chair, hands placed by your hips on the seat

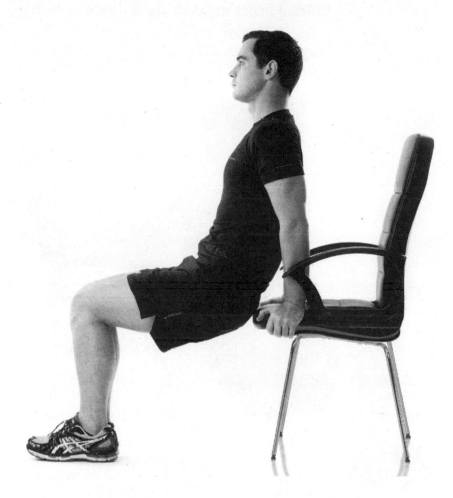

edge, feet flat on ground, away from body as far as possible

- Lift bum off and out from seat, bend elbows and lower towards ground

- Extend arms until straight again

- Do 20 reps, three sets.

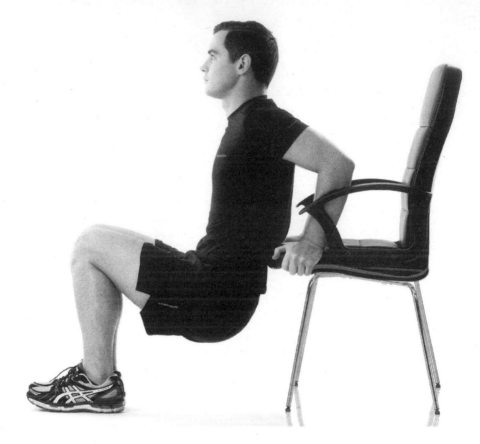

• **Wall press-ups:** *Simple to do and great for your shoulders too.*

- Bring thumbs and index fingers

of both hands together, creating a triangle between the hands

- Stand around two feet out from the wall

- Bend arms out to the side as you lean your body towards the wall, keeping

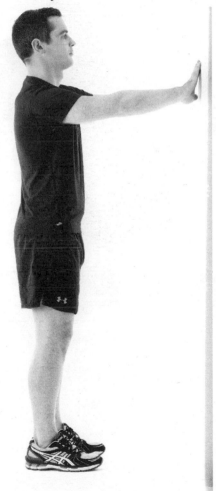

your back straight. BE CAREFUL NOT
TO APPROACH THE WALL TOO FAST

- Lock arms back out to starting
  position. If you feel any pain in your
  wrists simply bring the hands a little
  bit wider apart

- Do 20 reps, three sets.

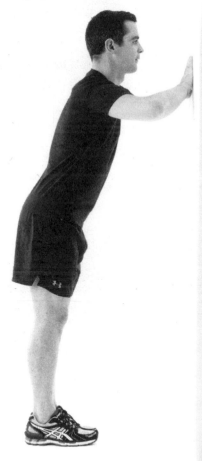

LEVEL TWO

- **Triceps press behind neck:** *You'll need a weight for each hand.*

    - Stand tall

    - Hold a weight or large bottle of water in each hand above your head, elbows by the ears

    - Bend arms and lower weight behind head until you reach base of neck

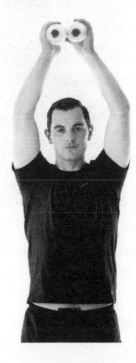

- Straighten arms back to the starting position. Squeeze your arms on the way up to give your triceps an extra little kick

- Do 20 reps, three sets.

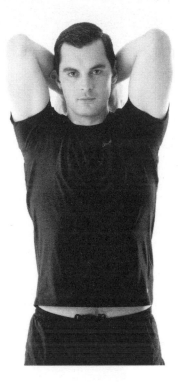

- **Lying triceps extensions**: *You'll need a weight for each hand.*

  - Lie on floor on your back, knees bent

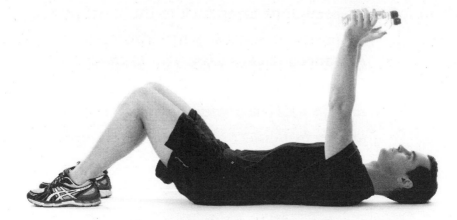

- With a weight in each hand, place arms straight out in front of you

- Bend at the elbow, with the weights coming slowly to the side of your face

- Straighten arms back out. Again remember to squeeze the back of your arms on the way up

- Do 20 reps, three sets.

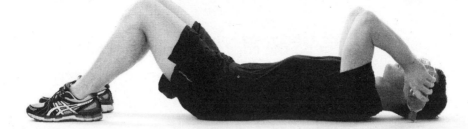

LEVEL THREE

- **Advanced triceps dips:** *The toughest but most effective of the BW exercises. The same as level one triceps dip except it's made tougher by flexing heels and resting on them.*

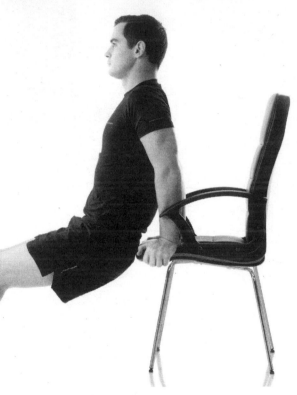

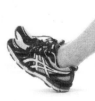

- Sit on the edge of a bench or chair, hands placed by your hips on the seat edge, feet flat on ground, away from body as far as possible

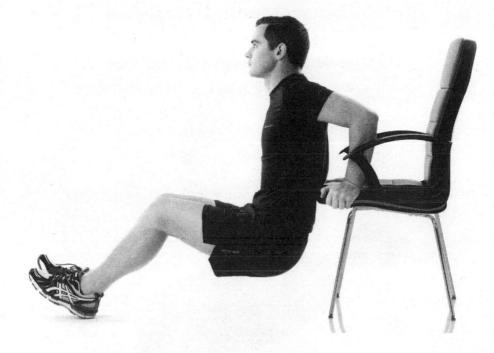

- Lift bum off and out from seat, bend elbows and lower towards ground

- Hold bum off floor for five seconds

- Extend arms until straight again

- Do 20 reps, three sets.

- **Tricep kickbacks:** *An old-school favourite of mine. You'll need a pair of weights.*

  - Stand tall, feet together, straight back. Hold a weight or bottle of water in each hand

  - Bend at your hips until back is parallel to floor

  - Extend arms out parallel to the floor

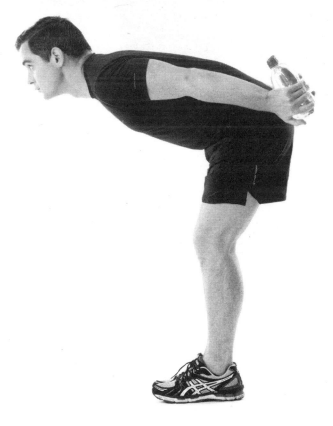

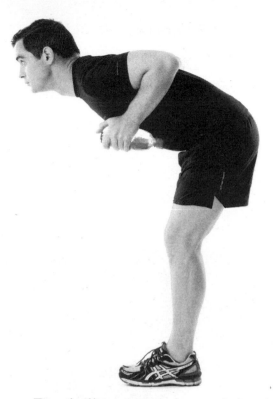

- Bend elbows to bring weights in towards your chest

- Push arms away from body.

- To maximise effect, push the weights up towards the ceiling.

- Do 20 reps, three sets.

**CARDIO AND RESISTANCE COMBINED MAKE
A GREAT TEAM**

If walking or running for your BTBW 1/3 cardio routine, consider introducing the stand-up exercises from these routines – they will work really well together.

6

FORGET ME AT YOUR PERIL! THE BTBW STRETCHES

'I could not believe the difference it made to introduces stretches to the end of my workout – getting out of bed the following day, waiting for the aches and pains, there was nothing. Had I really been putting myself through that for nothing, all those weeks?' – Sarah

I know, I know, you've finished your session, you're hungry and sweaty, and all you want to do is jump into the shower, then get a bite to eat! But what if I was to tell you that a few minutes – ok, no more than ten – will stop you from getting sore and stiff over the days following your workouts?

Over the course of an exercise session, the muscles of your body tighten up, leading to that painful sensation in your joints and muscles which you notice most often upon getting up the following day. We've all been there, right? However, integrating just a few minutes of stretches after a workout eliminates this by loosening out those tight muscles and boosting circulation to the area, reducing the build up of lactic acid. Sounds good, doesn't it?

I tend not to recommend stretching at the start of a session as your body is cold and there is a higher risk of strain and injury – but if you want to stretch early before your session try to warm up your body a little first – for example by walking for two or three minutes – gaining some heat into the muscles, then stretch from there. This will help to keep you safe and injury-free.

. . . .

The key time to stretch, *never to be missed*, is when you come in from your session. Combine this with the right post-session food and you are on your way to recovering to the optimum effect!

. . . .

So, here are the stretches. Ideally you should devote between five and ten minutes to these.

UPPER BODY STRETCHES

- **Hand and forearm stretch**

    - Stand with feet shoulder-width apart to give you balance

    - Bring hands to the front of your body and interlink fingers

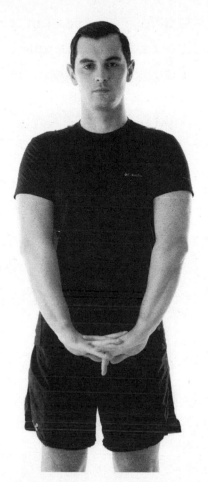

- Reverse hands and flex palms towards the floor

- If this is easy, raise your arms towards the front of your body, and flex hands away from you

- To take the stretch even farther, bring

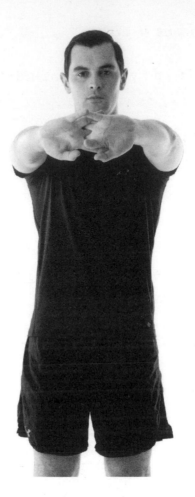

arms above head and flex hands toward sky. This is one of the best stretches I have come across for the arms, wrists and hands. Take it easy with this one and just progress as you feel comfortable.

- **Triceps stretch**

  - Stand with feet shoulder-width apart to give you balance

  - Raise right hand up into the air with left hand by side

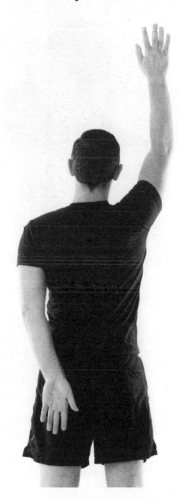

- Bend back elbow towards your back

- Bring left hand towards the middle of back, between shoulder blades,

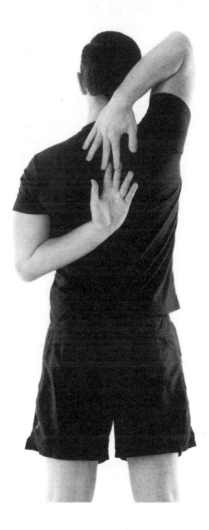

and try to bring right hand down to meet it

- Interlink hands if you can

- Change your arms so you start with your left hand in the air.

Note: If you find that you can't touch your hands, use a towel, moving hands down the towel as you become more flexible.

- **Shoulder stretch:** *Some basic shoulder rolls will do perfectly here.*

  - Stand with feet shoulder-width apart to give you balance

  - With hands by sides, relax neck and back

  - Roll shoulders back by making big circles backwards with your arms, aiming to get as deep a stretch as possible

  - Do five backwards, then five forwards, making nice slow, big circles, easing out the tension of the shoulders and neck.

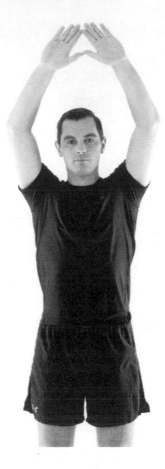

LOWER BODY STRETCHES

- **Quad stretch:** *Your quads are at the front of your leg above your knee, they form a large muscle group that loves to be stretched.*

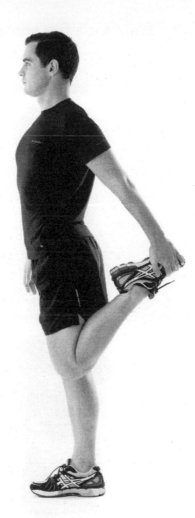

- Stand with feet together, beside a wall or a chair for support

- Take right ankle with right hand and pull ankle up towards your bum

- Hold for a few seconds, then change sides.

Note: Keep your knees together or as close as you can and stand tall so that your posture isn't affected.

- **Hamstring stretch:** *The hamstrings are at the back of the leg and run pretty much from your bum to your ankles.*

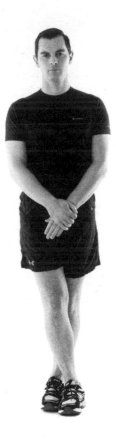

- Sit on floor

- Keep right leg straight and bring left leg in so that the sole of your shoe is by the inside of your right knee

- Take a deep breath in and stretch from your hips to try to touch the toes of your right foot. If you can't touch your toes use a Dyna Band or towel. Place the towel/band around the foot and take the two sides in your hands and gently pull yourself

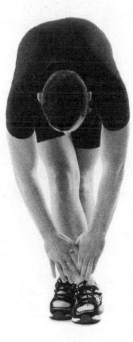

towards your foot. Over the course of time you will be able to do this without any assistance at all!

- Do the same stretch with left leg, taking it nice and easy. Take a break in between each side if you feel you need it.

• **Inner-leg stretch:** *The inner part of your leg can get sore from time to time after certain sessions, so this stretch will help you out.*

- Sit on floor with knees bent so the soles of your feet are together.

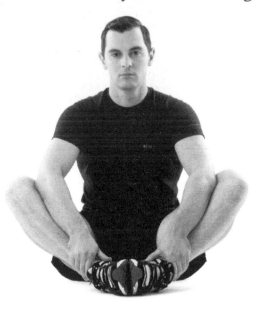

Place hands on feet and elbows on side of legs

- Push inside of legs out by placing pressure on legs with your elbows

- To apply more pressure, just put more effort into the elbows and you will feel a much greater stretch.

BACK STRETCHES

- **Cobra stretch:** *This is a classic stretch that takes its name from yoga.*

  - Lie on stomach with hands palms down by your shoulders to the side of your body

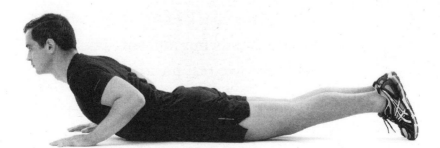

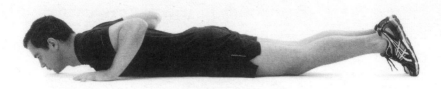

- Gently roll your body up off the floor using your hands for support – be careful not to push back too much, just ease back at your own pace

- Hold the stretch and then slowly lower your body down to the floor again.

• **Passive rest stretch:** *Wonderful for easing out lower-back strain.*

- Kneel on floor

- Lower bum back onto your heels and stretch hands out in front. This is the ideal passive rest position

- With each exhalation try to stretch hands farther out and get your bum lower onto your ankles

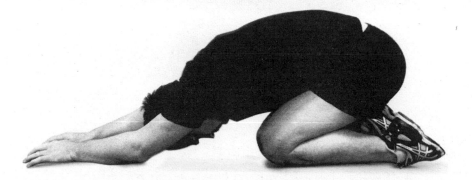

- If feet or ankles are sore, simply place your feet wider apart to make it more comfortable.

- **Cat pose:** *A classic pose to loosen out strains in your lower, mid and even upper spine.*

  - Go on all fours. Ensure that hands and knees are shoulder-width apart and that you are totally relaxed

  - Take a deep breath in and pull your belly button up towards your spine

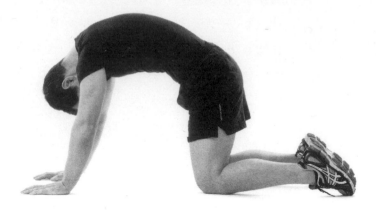

- Inhale as you curl spine up just like a cat would do (hence the name)

- Breathe out as you relax your back and let your stomach return towards floor

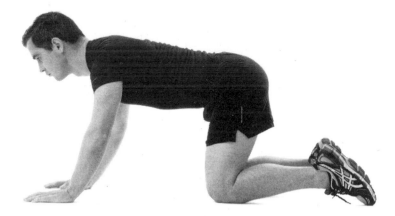

- Aim for between five and ten of these, gathering any stress and tension in the back on the breath in, and releasing and relaxing the back on the breath out.

TIPS

- **How long to hold for:** With most of the stretches I would aim to hold for twenty to thirty seconds to get the maximum benefit out of the stretch. Ease into it and as you begin to feel your body loosening out, you can then push it a little farther and deeper into the stretch – but be careful not to push it too far.

- **How many to do:** This depends on how you feel, but as a rule of thumb you should devote at least ten minutes to stretching after your workout. Depending on the intensity of your workout, I would certainly recommend between two and three sets as I feel that this is where you get the maximum benefit.

- **Before or after your workout?** After all the way! But remember, if you do want to stretch beforehand make sure you have warmed up a little before you do anything to ensure that you stay injury and strain free.

- **Dyna-Bands:** These can help you to stretch farther and push your body a little farther – though a large towel folded up will do exactly the same job for you. Be careful not to stretch too far or too much by using these – if it's painful, stop. Stretching should be about easing back and enjoying the session.

THE EASIEST AND ULTIMATE DE-STRESSER

We all get days where stress gets the better of us. You feel like tearing your hair out and lose the ability to focus on work, life or pretty much anything. You would do anything to get rid of the stress and get back the ability to focus; well the good news is that this simple method is the fastest, cheapest and easiest way to de-stress you will ever find! Follow these quick and easy steps:

- Find a quiet space for a few minutes and either sit, stand or lie on the floor

- Close your eyes and focus on your breathing, taking a deep breath in and deep breath out

- Now as you breathe in, I want you to hold your breath for ten seconds. For these ten seconds, tense all the muscles in the legs as hard as you can, taking all the stress and tension that is in them. After the ten seconds breathe out, releasing everything you feel tightening in your legs. Repeat this three times, each time relaxing more and more as you begin to chill

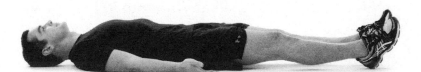

- Now repeat the same process for your upper body, breathing in and tensing your arms, chest, back and neck while holding your breath for ten seconds

- Now return to just focus on your breathing. Take your time and open your eyes whenever you feel ready to face the world again

- You don't have to repeat this three times, it can be as many as you feel you need to get the tension out.

7
Q&A THE BTBW WAY

I get asked the same questions time and again, and here I've compiled a list of them so that you don't need to. We've touched upon some of these points in the book, but it's no harm to recap.

Q: Will weights make me overly muscular?

A: No, they certainly won't! By doing light weights with high repetitions, you will simply tone your body muscle, adding to your lean body mass. This helps to give you shape, structure and tone. Being skinny and soft is no fun at all, why not aim to be slim and firm? This is what the weights will do for you.

. . . .

Q: How do protein-only diets work and do you recommend them?

A: Protein-only diets force the body to eat

away at its own fat stores, something that's also known as ketosis, and it is this process that causes the bad breath and bad skin associated with protein-only diets. Generally, this is the most common type of diet on the market and can give short-term, fast results. However, as a long-term option, I don't advise it for both reasons of sustainability and health. A balanced diet needs good carbs, simple as.

· ·

Q: Will running only help me lose weight?

A: Any form of exercise that burns more calories that you have taken in will help you lose weight. But it should never be the aim of any exercise routine to simply lose weight – and running alone will not give you the improved muscle tone you are looking for. But it will be perfect as part of an overall training plan, just like the one I have used in this book.

· ·

Q: What are heart-rate monitors all about?

A: Heart-rate monitors are the straps that go under your bust line, and relate information to a watch on your wrist. This information will tell you how hard you are working in your session, just like a rev counter in your car. Your body burns different fuel depending on how hard you are working and this is what the heart-rate monitor will tell you. This is why they are so useful when you are training, especially if you find that you have hit a weight-loss plateau – which normally means that you aren't working hard enough in your sessions. A heart-rate monitor will help to ensure that you are.

. . . .

Q: How do I get over my fear of gyms?

A: This is a common issue because so many gyms are big, unfriendly spaces with grunting muscle-bound men. So let me demystify them for you. Most gyms are made up of three areas: cardio, resistance and stretching. It is important to be a consumer and talk to the gym staff, push them to engage with you and give you a programme, show you how the machines work and change your programme every few weeks. Sometimes all you have to do is ask and once you strike up a relationship with the staff, they will look out for you when you are in the gym.

. . . .

Q: I get de-motivated easily, how can I change this?

A: Sometimes the bigger picture can seem overwhelming. Our final goal can feel too far away from where we are now and, after an initial enthusiastic burst, the shine of our new routine begins to wear off. That is why it's really important to think in small steps, and set small goals and rewards.

. . . .

Focus on what you have set yourself to do this day, and this day only! Then set about doing that, and nothing more.

. . . .

Congratulate yourself for your work, especially on days when you least feel like it. Remind yourself regularly: results are not immediate, but take heart from every extra minute you add to your routine that seemed impossible a few days or a week before.

Fitness is incremental and remember that a slow steady pace means the best for long-term results. Which means the end of fad diets, quick fixes, yo-yo weight gain and loss, and all the psychological baggage that goes with it. The BTBW Plan is about life-change, and just like life, it can have its ups and downs – but by being realistic and honest with yourself from the start, setting realistic, achievable goals based on the information in these pages, and staying mindful of the fact that every step on the way is a building block towards a new you, you will be much less likely to let de-motivation get the better of you.

. . . .

Q: How soon will I see results?

A: You will begin to notice a difference within seven days, particularly if you're making the changeover from a poor diet heavy in white carbs and refined foods. Within two weeks you will see noticeable differences in your clothes and by week three, your friends will be telling you how amazing you look. But remember just how important the food you eat is – if you're not making the changes to your food intake, the results that you see won't be as good.

. . . .

Q: I only want a flat tummy, can I concentrate just on that?

A: Concentrating on one area of the body in this way is called spot-reducing. But technically speaking, it's actually impossible, as isolating one area can't really be done without improving the other body parts around that area too. And besides, an all-over tone in your body is what you should be aiming for – it looks better aside from being better for you! So stick to the overall BTBW Plan is my advice.

....

Q: Should I wear make-up in the gym or when I train?

A: Ideally not. Your skin needs to be able to breathe and by covering it with make-up, you are preventing this. Working up a sweat is actually good for you as it helps the body to eliminate toxins from your system. So next time you go to the gym, make-up off and let your body sweat!

....

Q: I hate running – can you help me?

A: You don't have to run if you don't want to. People are constantly taking up running to lose weight and this is the wrong reason. You should only take up running if you actually want to run. You won't last long trying to do something you don't like, we all know that! Having said that, very few people love running when they start it. It's hard work that the body isn't used to, and it's easy to convince ourselves that it isn't for us.

. . . .

My advice is to give it at least two weeks before you decide. What often happens is that as a routine becomes established and the body gets used to it, people who thought they hated running discover that quite the opposite is true.

. . . .

However, if you've tried all that and still just don't like it, it's possible it isn't for you. Luckily, there are many other sports out there that you will actually enjoy so why not try to find one of those instead? Making exercise fun is half the battle.

. . . .

Q: Am I heavier when I have my period?

A: Yes, no question about it. Fluid retention before and after your period can be anything between three and seven pounds. You should always take this into consideration when you do your regular weigh-ins – it is something that so many people forget about and can lead to serious de-motivation. The good news is that the healthier you are, the lower any difficult physical effects around the time of your period will be. You will have less stomach pain and bloating – that on its own is a serious motivator to get fit! And clients frequently report to me a lessening in pre-menstrual tension as a result of regular exercise, too!

. . . .

Q: Should I tell my friends I am trying to lose weight?

A: No! The more people you tell, the harder it will be as you are putting more and more pressure on yourself. And it's nice to be told you look great by people who don't know you are trying to lose weight – it acts as a great motivator. So my advice is you tell as few people as possible, knuckle down and get the work done, lose weight yourself and enjoy the compliments when they come!

. . . .

Q: Should I bother with a sports bra?

A: As I've said, sports bras are an essential piece of kit when it comes to training. They help to keep your chest moving as little as possible, making it more comfortable for you to train and also helping to protect your back as well, as there is less movement going on. There are so many different brands on the market I would just recommend trying them out until you find one that is the most comfortable for you. The less movement you feel, the better the job your sports bra is doing for you!

· ·

Q: I've tried every diet going, nothing has worked – can you help me?

A: Diet alone is never the best method to lose weight and keep it off, and short-term, radical weight-loss plans lead to short-term results. The first step you need to take is to rethink the very basics of what a diet is. Rather than seeing it as something you do to lose weight, see it for what it is: a way of life. A proper healthy diet, coupled with regular exercise, are the only tools you will ever need to lose weight, and keep it off. And there's nothing faddish about that.

And that's what the BTBW Food Plan is all about.

. . . .

Q: I don't want to give up alcohol, do I have to?

A: I discuss this in more detail in the Food Plan section, but in short, the good news is, you don't have to. Remember, I am never going to recommend anything that is too strict as most people won't stick to it. Once you tell yourself you can't have something, it becomes the only thing you want. I would say keep alcohol in your life, but cut back and only drink one day a week. Certainly cut out the beers and ciders, but you can have spirits or wine. The latter are better quality and will have less of an effect on your waistline and you'll feel less bloated! By not aiming to cut it out totally, you are making a lifetime plan that will ensure you stay healthy for life.

. . . .

Q: How can I find the time? It's impossible!

A: Not being able to find the time is never a good excuse! No matter how busy your day, how crazy your life, there is always time to exercise. It could be fifteen minutes walking four times a day or it could only be one session per week, but regardless of what it is, it all helps. More often than not, it is just a matter of prioritising your health, putting yourself first. Take out your diary, schedule in your training, your weekly shop and any other health-based time. Once it is there, stick to it – do not move it. No matter what happens, you must keep to your diary and work everything else around it.

Ask yourself tough questions. How much time do you spend in front of the telly in the evening? Or out socialising? If you can create the time for these things, you can create the time for exercise. It's all about setting priorities. And pretty soon, you'll want to. If you really want to do it, if you really have the right goals, you will put yourself first.

. . . .

Q: Where do I start? I get scared thinking about it.

A: Don't worry, this book will guide you through everything you need to know. Start with your goals, create your BTBW Plan, start eating the BTBW way, start exercising. All the tools you will ever need are here, thcy are exactly the same tools that I give my clients and now you have them too. I have taken out all the confusion for you, all the scary words, to give you the real information, the important information, the information that will get you the results you want.

. . . .

Q: What if it's too hard?

A: If you are finding it too hard, it means that you are pushing yourself too hard at the start. Remember that Rome wasn't built in a day, you need to start slow and steadily build it up as you get stronger. Start gently, gradually increase your workouts and your walks or runs. Remember the talk test tool I gave you – if you can't talk in any of your workouts, you are working far too hard. So build it up gradually, enjoy the feeling of getting fitter and stronger as you see yourself progress each week.

. . . .

Q: What if I fall off the wagon? That's what always happens.

A: Like so many people, you are a yoyo exerciser. You try all the quick fixes, until now. You won't have a wagon to fall off anymore as this is no quick fix. The tools in this book will lead you to lifelong health, by creating balance. Keeping your favourite foods but modified to their healthier incarnation – wholefood – and in moderation. Educating you with all the information you need to make informed choices so you don't fall for the quick fixes that advertisers bombard you with each January.

. . . .

Q: Will I be sore?

A: Whenever we activate muscle groups that have been dormant, there is a certain amount of discomfort. When you exercise, you are stretching your muscle fibres, creating minute tears. Over the course of time these become stronger and firmer, creating that tone that you want – but it's not entirely painless. But by easing into your new routine gently, you will reduce the amount of pain you feel. Work too hard and you will be very, very sore for a few days, try to avoid this by not doing too much on day one!

· ·

Q: Why am I more sore two days later?

A: This is called DOMS, or Delayed Onset Muscle Soreness. The muscle adaptation takes some time causing this soreness. You can reduce this by improving your food and using the techniques to recover, the most obvious one being stretching, which we've covered. By improving your recovery techniques, you will be reducing the amount of pain you will be feeling. As your body gets fitter, you will begin to recover faster, to the point where you can train hard and will have no soreness the following day at all, though it takes time to get to this point.

. . . .

Q: How can I stop it?

A: You can reduce the amount of pain by stretching after your workouts and using simple recovery methods, such as a hot Epsom salts bath and massage. Using simple stretches, like the ones in the Chapter 6, at the end of your workout will help reduce muscle damage. The Epsom salts will help to relax the muscles and eliminate lactic acid from the muscle tissue. Massage will help you to improve the circulation in the area and relieve any aches or strains – it's also a fantastic way to relax your mind.

. . . .

Q: What is this cold bath talk all about?

A: Using cold water as a muscle relaxant is possibly the best way to relieve muscle pain and aches, though it's not to everyone's liking. Ideally a quick dip in the sea would do it as you are getting cold and salts into your muscles. The cold helps to reduce lactic acid build-up and improve circulation. If you don't live by the sea, a cold shower or cold bath is perfect. Grin and bear it for as long as you can. The good news is that there is research to prove that cold showers/baths can help to speed up weight loss as well as recovery. So not only are you helping your body to recover, you are also helping to increase your weight loss too.

8

GETTING IN GEAR FOR THE BTBW PLAN

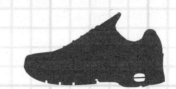

'Fancy, 'super-duper' runners do not make running easier so I went and got free advice in a sports store and didn't pay a fortune for the correct pair of runners for me. My sports bra wasn't giving enough support so I solved that problem with and secret support T-shirt.' – Gemma

Getting fit is rewarding and takes a lot of hard work – so why not enjoy all that work by picking the coolest and best gear for what you are doing? And it doesn't have to cost the earth. The next few pages will give you all you need to know about pretty much anything that you are looking to buy over the coming months and years.

RUNNERS

Assuming you already own a pair of runners, you need to first make sure they are up to the job. Inspect the soles. They should be evenly worn. Most people wear out more on one side or the other, depending if you 'pronate' or 'supinate' when you walk. If they are very uneven, you'll need to replace them. The second thing you need to look for is how worn down the rubber is, if it is worn down to the white of the runner, again, you'll need to replace them.

Now turn your attention to the absorption system within the runner, which is generally placed at the back or the side of the runners. Place your thumb just under it and try to press it in. Give it a good squeeze. If you can press it easily then it's time for a change, as the system has seen better days. Also look for cracks or breaks around this area, all signs for change.

Finally, if you have just put your runners in the washing machine, then I have some bad news for you, you will be needing to change them too. The washing machine process, regardless of temperature, will also damage the absorption system. It may make them white and shiny, but it will also make the runners more prone to smelling badly too, which is never good!

If you have seen that your runners need to be changed, what can you do to ensure you get the best pair that suits you?

Gone are the days of buying runners off the shelf. Now when you buy, ask to have your gait checked. This just means checking how you walk or run to ensure that you are getting into the best runner to suit your foot type. There are several shops that offer this service for free all year round and once you do it once you won't need to do it again. It is essential to do to ensure your feet are in the best runners possible, which is not necessarily the most expensive – something that's always good!

If you are running on a regular basis, ideally you should look at changing your runners every four to six months, if you are walking regularly then you should be getting a little longer out of them. Remember to keep checking your runners every month using the tips above and you will be confident that your runners are keeping your feet and joints safe and sound.

With new runners, blisters can be a problem, so before you follow that surge of determination and head out for a long run, think first! There are several things you can do to avoid blisters and chafing from new runners. The first is to wear them only for short runs for the first week or two, then gradually increase your distance in the new runners. It is amazing how even experienced runners forget this blister-beware rule! If you find that you are still getting chafing then apply some Vaseline to the affected areas, just a little, rub in deeply and this should solve the problem. If you're still getting blisters even after both of these top tips, then try loosening the laces a little, but to be honest you shouldn't have any problems once you increase the distance you run gradually.

TOPS

There are many brands on the market, with different fits and styles to suit all body types. I always recommend that my clients try out various brands until they find one that suits them best, because it's different for everyone. I do advise that you steer clear of pure cotton fabrics, as these will increase your sweat rate, which can lead to discomfort from chafing around the body. Look for fabrics such as Dri-Fit, or basically any half-Lycra synthetic fabric, as these will make your runs and workouts so much more enjoyable – and the more comfortable you feel, the longer you are likely to exercise.

You should certainly have a really good rain jacket too. For walking, a more expensive hardshell jacket may be required to give you more wind proofing as well as keep you dry, but these tend to be too heavy for running. Runners should have a lightweight rain jacket, which will keep you dry but also allow your body to breathe. I love luminous colours as not only do they look good, they also help people see you on the road, keeping you safe all year round.

SOCKS

The same rule applies to socks as to tops: leave the heavy cotton fabrics behind. Go for the synthetic mixture as they will help keep your feet dry and comfortable. For a longer-looking calf and leg, go for the ankle socks, just make sure they offer you enough protection at the back of the heel to avoid blisters. There are so many different brands on the market that you can take your choice depending on your budget – the important thing is the fabric.

BRAS

Ok, I can't claim to have personal experience in this department, but I do know it's seriously important for women to find the best sports bra possible. You want a bra that reduces movement in your chest as much as possible. This will not only help your chest keep its shape, it will also help to reduce the amount of pressure placed upon your back and posture. The bigger your chest, the more pressure is placed on your back, neck and shoulders – and the more important your sports bra choice. Shop around, try different brands and see which one suits you best.

MUSIC

Some clients I have love to work out to dance music, others to classical. There's no best option, it is whatever you prefer. Your subconscious mind will increase your tempo when you listen to high-speed dance music, especially when you are running or doing a high-intensity workout. The important part, in my opinion, is that if music keeps you exercising longer and gives you a better session, then you should be using it.

I always recommend you leave the phone behind when exercising – why put yourself in the way of distraction? Remember that your session is *your* time, away from the stresses of daily life, from work and family commitments, time to push your body and get the most out of your workout. If you have your phone, you'll only be tempted to take calls or answer texts – or these days even check your email!

For those days that you really do not feel like starting your session, I strongly recommend you create what I call an emergency playlist of tunes that you like and know will get you psyched up. It's easier to put on music than start a workout, right? But your emergency playlist will give you the boost you need to get you off the couch, out on the road or into the gym or your home exercise space to do your BTBW routine.

DUMBBELLS

In terms of equipment for your BTBW Plan, all you will really need are a pair of dumbbells – and two full 500ml water bottles will even suffice starting out. These can provide a workout for any body part, without the expense of machines or gym memberships. There are many different types to choose from, but I would normally advise against the chrome interchangeable ones as they tend to be awkward and slightly bigger. The plastic-or velour-covered dumbbells are normally easier and more comfortable to use and can be bought for as little as twenty euro from most sports shops around the country. In terms of weight, 2-kilogram dumbbells are normally a great start, though if you haven't exercised for a long time maybe start with the 1.5-kilogram ones.

EXERCISE MATS

There are many different colours and types on the market. The key thing to consider when choosing is the anti-slip function. Rubber compounds tend to work better and stick to the floor better than anything else. Most yoga mats are made with rubber compounds and roll up small so that you don't waste storage space, so these make a good choice.

WATCHES

A watch is a crucial part of getting fit, and it is something that I have to recommend you invest in. No matter how fit you are, a watch will help you to set goals and push yourself that little bit harder.

If you can stretch to around a hundred euro, you will be able to get a watch with a GPS function, now you are really talking! GPS watches will give you your speed and distance for your workouts, ensuring that you really are getting the most out of the session. They are simple to use and will turn your workouts around instantly, as there is nowhere to hide when the statistics are directly in front of you, glaring at you guiltily. I have used Garmin watches for years and find them to be reliable and effective, but there are many brands out there. They range in price from one hundred to four hundred euro, but the more expensive ones normally just have functions that you won't really use, no matter how cool they sound.

9

BTBW FIRST-HAND: THE SUCCESS STORIES

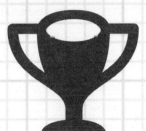

JANE'S STORY

My entire adult life I've been unhappy with my weight. I felt it was somehow out of my control as I found losing weight so unbelievably hard, all-consuming and torturous that I would have paid someone to do it for me.

I tried every diet imaginable from cabbage soup or no carbs to diet shakes and calorie-counting, but found sticking to something consistently so difficult. I could be very disciplined with food during the week, then after a night out at the weekend, I would nurse my hangover with anything I wanted. The cycle would continue with punishment on a Monday, cutting out a food group or spurred from guilt start a fad diet in desperation – it was truly miserable, erratic, cruel and fruitless.

When I did lose weight, compliments from others would encourage me to celebrate or treat myself with … food! Eventually bringing me right back to where I started. I was in constant yo-yo.

The day I met Karl for my consultation, my life changed – sounds cheesy but it is completely true. We discussed some goals. First on my list was a half-marathon in Connemara, I explained my absolute dreams in terms of weight, clothes size, fitness, etc. Karl advised me on food, portion control, exercise and my running training. I met with Karl weekly and his excitement and enthusiasm made me want to do better and helped keep me motivated. Karl spurred on my own motivation and desire to make a change. It has been the most amazing journey and experience for me – the best investment I have ever made in myself. In four months I went from struggling to run for a couple of minutes to running a half-marathon, I have lost 24 pounds, almost 30 inches of fat and am now the proud owner of a size 8 body – which is the right size for my frame.

For all the years I struggled with my weight, I look back on my four-month transformation and it was so easy, exciting and genuinely enjoyable in comparison. Switching to a realistic manageable food diet and crucially incorporating exercise means I enjoy all of life's indulgences now – just in a balanced way. Exercise is now a massive part of my routine, and I couldn't be without it. I love working hard, enjoy the satisfaction after working up a good sweat and am relishing in feeling fit. I feel like a new person and so full of energy.

A desire to change combined with a fitness goal of doing a half-marathon shifted my entire focus from dropping pounds to something so much more exciting. The feeling after completing a 10K run when you know you couldn't have done it five weeks previously is amazing. My hard work has paid off, my life has changed, it has spurred others around me to do the same and I feel very lucky and happy to be where I am today.

MIRANDA'S STORY

How do you start a story that spans over thirty-three years? I have been overweight for as long as I can remember.

I have found it hard to find clothes to fit me from a young age. Spent most of my life listening to people saying, 'She's a fine child, sure she's big boned.' I always played camogie from a young age and I think that helped to keep the weight at bay a little bit. That was until I started secondary school and started to socialise. I think that was when it really hit home that while all my friends could wear the nice dresses, I was finding it impossible to find tops and jeans to fit, never mind a dress. On a night out, I always felt on the outside of the circle looking at all the girls in their fantastic new dresses. Of course I was the typical jovial, fat person.

I've known my husband most of my life as he was a childhood friend. So my weight never came into question. He always took me for the person I was. Every year around the 1st of January, I would start a weight-loss programme and for a while I stuck to it rigidly. I would walk every evening and the food I ate was healthy. Like everything with me, nothing lasted forever and I once again became a couch potato. The diet went out the window and was replaced by pints of cider and Chinese food.

Over the years, I have tried many diets from Weight Watchers to Motivation Clinics but without any great success. I have listened to all sorts of comments about my weight. One year while on holidays in sunny Spain, to reach the beach from the apartment I had to go down three flights of stairs. Going down was fine but having to come back up was a nightmare. I was breathless and had to stop several times.

On my return from holidays, I decided it was now or never. I needed to do something about my weight. Around this time *Operation Transformation* started. I decided I would pick a leader and follow their plan. I listened attentively to the advice of Karl Henry and the other member of the team. By the time the programme finished, I had lost a stone. I decided I needed a mentor and a personal trainer. I rang Karl and he invited me to Dublin for a consultation. That was three years ago and Karl has helped to motivate me, keep me focused and above all determined to lose weight.

I am now four stone four pounds lighter, self-confident and I can complete a 10K run without effort. My long-term goal is to complete a half-marathon. I am not a fast runner by any standard, I will be completing it for myself.

Without the support of my family and Karl my mentor I would not be fit and healthy today.

I know I will never put the weight back on. I love my new clothes too much – and the compliments that people give me.

GEMMA'S STORY

Why do I run?

Jealousy, pure unadulterated jealousy …

Sitting in the car watching runners out and about – some alone deep in their thoughts, some with music, some out with friends chatting and all of them content. I suppose I was jealous of their freedom more than their fitness. I could see contentment in their faces, focus in their eyes and effortless drive to carry on. I loved sports and have played many but never conquered running … pain in my chest, burning in my throat, feeling that my lungs were about to explode out of my chest, sore legs, sore back, blistered feet – the list was endless and I let it get the better of me every time until … no more, I was going to learn to love running. I wanted that freedom.

I approached a friend who I would see out running and asked her to come out with me for a while until I got the hang of it. We started walking and adding periods of running into the walks until a slow jog became easier than a fast walk. We would go for a slow jog a couple of times a week and stayed out for longer and longer as the weeks

222

went by. We mostly went together, but it didn't always suit and the runs on my own were harder. I had to have music in my ears to drown out the sound of my much-laboured breathing.

Nine months into running, it wasn't getting any easier and I thought back to those people that inspired me and wondered how long I had to do this to get what they had. Some days, the thoughts of a run put me in a foul mood, some runs I looked forward to were awful from start to finish … So do I give up or see if I can get over this and start enjoying this running business?

I started talking to other runners and soon discovered that eating no less than two hours before I ran sorted out my IBS. Fancy, 'super-duper' runners do not make running easier so I went and got free advice in a sports store and didn't pay a fortune for the correct pair of runners for me. My sports bra wasn't giving enough support so I solved that problem with a secret support T-shirt. Skipping stretching does more harm than good and music only distracts from getting that focus and freedom I longed for. Setting a goal helps with getting a routine going so I decided to do a half-marathon and used Karl's plan to train for it.

I've done the half-marathon now and it was during that training that it all seemed to come together for me. It turns out running is not easy, it takes a lot of time, effort and commitment to even begin to enjoy it and it takes discipline to keep it up.

It's eighteen months later and I love it. Running has given me all that I thought it would and so much more. It gives me time to process the day, solve the problems, come up with answers and make plans. Every run, love it or hate it, blows off the cobwebs, gives a sense of achievement and brings renewed energy for the next one.

AUDREY'S STORY

I am a thirty-seven-year-old single mother. I met my daughter's father through my workplace. After a few weeks he asked me out and we started dating. Within a few months, I was pregnant. We moved in together but slowly everything changed. During my pregnancy, I was starting to feel isolated as he would always go out but I always had to stay in. I had my daughter in May 1997, and after that everything started to go wrong. A few months later, things were taken out of my hands and I had to split up with him because our relationship was affecting my mental health and my relationship with my family. It was hard, but it had to be done for my own sanity and the safety of my daughter – but it left me with no self-confidence or self-esteem.

My weight started to fly up as there was just the two of us. It was easier to get takeaways after work instead of cooking. I started many diets – Weight Watchers, Unislim – but could only ever stick to them for a few months. Whatever I lost, I always put it back on plus a few extra pounds and eventually gave up again.

One Sunday morning at work, I had to look back on Saturday's security footage. Who was that person wearing my clothes!

It was me! Only four times bigger than I thought I was – my immediate reaction was to delete the footage. I couldn't bear to look at that person in front of me. During my tea break, while munching through my second packet of crisps, I decided enough was enough. Time to look after myself, lose the weight and get back the person that I was all those years ago – find myself again, the confident, outgoing active person I was.

In February 2009, my sister and I decided to do something about our weight so we rang Karl. I found Mr Henry and replaced Mr Tayto – and I haven't looked back since.

My first encounter with Karl was a cold one. It was snowing outside. My fitness test was a disaster. I couldn't run for five minutes and I was out of breath and dizzy. I got a fitness plan and a food plan that changed my whole concept on life. I can now run 10K and survive. Previously I couldn't run up the stairs without feeling like I had just climbed the Devil's Bit. I now eat fruit and vegetables that I didn't know existed. I was allergic to healthy living. I was bitten by the exercise bug and I have gone from XL Spanx to exercise pants.

After our first consultation, my sister and I decided to set goals which kept us challenged and focused. I now train at least five times a week, between running on the roads and going to the gym. I ran my first 5K in the Phoenix Park. It was tough and I had to run and walk a little bit but I was getting closer to the finish line where Karl was on the lines encouraging me to keep going. That was three years ago and since then I have run 5K and 10K runs from start to finish, improving my previous times. I have now entered a half-marathon in the Phoenix Park which I am determined to complete. After that I will re-evaluate my fitness levels and maybe setting my goals even higher – maybe a full marathon next year. I am now 3½ stone lighter and my fitness levels are higher than what they were in my teens.

Now when I look back on footage in the shop, I can focus on the thieves and not myself, as I look five years younger and healthier than I did three years ago. I am now looking forward to a happier, healthier future.

Tús maith leath na hoibre (A good start is half the work).

SANDRA'S STORY

I was what some might call a 'big' girl, what Gok Wan might call 'curvy' and what I called 'a woman who needs to watch her weight – 24/7'. So when a friend asked me to be her bridesmaid, I thought it was time to take control and make sure that photo of me in the brown chiffon dress on her mother's wall was going to be one I'd look fondly on for years to come.

That was eight years ago and my first engagement with the concept of going to the gym. For the years that followed, I engaged in what I called the debit/credit technique of life. Knock back a few mojitos on a Saturday night after dinner with dessert and cheese, but that's OK because I've run ten miles today, right? I started running in July 2008 and after my first, tough 5 mile race of 50 minutes and 42 seconds I was bitten by the bug . . . and celebrated with an all-night session with my brothers and their friends! Since then I've run countless 5k, 10k, 5 mile and 10 mile runs, 6 half marathons, 1 marathon, gained a true appreciation of a fit and healthy body . . . and gained a stone in weight.

Over the years I'd gotten quite lazy with my attitude towards exercise. It became a means to an end. I knew I could eat junk if I just kept running and training. But eventually it had to catch up on me. Earlier this year, I was 12 stone 7 pounds. I wasn't visibly overweight as I'm tall so I could lie to myself that not much had changed, but my clothes confirmed to me every morning that, yes, I was indeed 12 stones 7 pounds. And every ounce of that weighed on my confidence, my motivation, my drive. I felt terrible, I hated my clothes and

I hated my body. Humorous, self-deprecating digs about my weight became the focus of every conversation I had with friends.

Then I got the call from Wedding Headquarters once again. I was invited to be chief bridesmaid for my dear friend whom I've known since we were 7. I was delighted to accept an opportunity to wear a pretty dress and witness my friend marry the man she loved. And then the reality set in. I was going to be the 35-year-old, single, 'heavy-set' bridesmaid – cue sympathetic sigh. Something had got to be done! It wasn't even just about the bridesmaid thing, it was everything! I needed to get a focus back, like myself again and remember all the good things about having a healthy mind and a healthy body.

So I went PT shopping and that's when I came across Karl. I knew of him but still I was going to interview this guy and make sure together we could deliver on what I wanted to achieve. This was serious stuff!

I arrived at Henry Headquarters on a wet May evening, shaking with nerves, feeling like I was going to a therapy session. How was I going to admit that I weighed 12 stone who-knows-how-many pounds, that I could go drink-for-drink with almost any guy, and often did, that two bars of chocolate a day had become the norm, but rest assured I also ran about three times a week? I needn't have worried. Karl met me, put me at ease, asked me lots of questions and reassured me that he knew where I was coming from, what I wanted to do and was going to guide and help me to get there. We talked about what my ultimate goal was, what I'd done in the past, what I liked and didn't like, what I ate, drank, didn't eat and didn't drink. We settled on two main goals: Longford Half Marathon this year in under 2 hours, a personal best (PB) for me, and 10 stone 13.9999999 pounds by the wedding at the beginning of August.

The next session was booked in and I was weighed and measured. The words were all a bit of a haze . . . 6.5 inches off your waist (that's over half a foot), 12 stone 2 pounds (at least I was going in the right direction) . . . inch off hips . . . off leg . . . off neck. It seemed like a lot of inches to lose, but I just kept thinking of that dress I had to fit into and less bulk to haul around Longford at the end of August.

Over the course of ten weeks we set weekly goals to achieve weight loss and build fitness. I'd always bought into the 'muscle weighs more than fat' myth so when I was training but not losing weight I assured myself that this was normal. So for me to achieve an increase in fitness and speed as well as a reduction in weight just helps me every week to hit my targets. I keep a food diary and send this to Karl along with details of my training. He gives me regular feedback and really helps to motivate me and keep me on track. I've always claimed determination is not my problem, it's focus and motivation and Karl supports me with that in bucket loads.

My friends all ask what diet I'm on, but it never feels like a diet in the old-school sense. I've made small but sensible changes to my eating, making clever decisions so as to never feel hungry or bloated. My one treat day a week has become something I carefully consider, weigh up the pros and cons of every option and thoroughly enjoy it, guilt-free! If you've ever, like me, wondered which could you live without, red wine or chocolate, then allow yourself one treat a week. There is no doubt you'll have the answer by the end of week one. For the record I can live without chocolate.

It's not always easy. There are days when I feel

like I'd murder a slice of chocolate cake, but what keeps me motivated is that picture in my head of the aubergine halter neck, fitted-waist bridesmaid dress and running across the finish line in Longford (not in the dress!) at a time of 1 hour 59 minutes and 59 seconds. And I realise that if I really want the chocolate cake, I can have it on Saturday as my treat.

I recently ran a 5 mile race in Dublin. Thirty minutes before the race started, I sat in my car with one of my friends who said to me 'Will we just go to the pub instead?'. I have never in my life been so tempted to spin the car around 180 degrees and hightail it to my local. I really did not want to do this race; I'd just flown home from holidays and had a lot of laundry in my living room. But I remembered I had a session with Karl the next day and had a lot of holiday 'baggage' so this run had to be done. At the start line I turned to my friend and said 'I'm just going to see how this goes, if I have to walk this, I'll walk.' 41 mins 44 seconds later I crossed the line. That was 3 minutes faster than my previous PB. I wondered was I mistaken, maybe delirious from my flight, but no, my watch confirmed what the clock said: 41:44. I never let myself believe before that anything below 44 minutes was possible, but I'd done it. I'd not only broken my PB, I'd smashed it. I was walking on air.

As I write this, my friend's wedding is this weekend and at last weigh in I was 10 stone 11.2 pounds, 6.5 inches smaller on my waist to add to all the other inches I've lost off my body. I am toned, fit and happy. I feel great mentally and physically. My confidence is back up and I like myself again. I set goals and targets and with the help of a super trainer I've achieved them. The bridesmaid's dress fits like a glove. My friends and family compliment the happy, slim, fit and toned me. I, rather embarrassingly, check out my trim waist in the bathrooms at work and smile excitedly. I have tone in places where I didn't even know I had muscles! I run at a consistent 9 minute mile pace now, I'm not taking walk breaks during my runs, I feel strong, challenged and fit. I will achieve that sub 2 hour half marathon and I know I will really, really enjoy the treat afterwards.

USEFUL STUFF

APPENDIX 1: THE A–Z OF RUNNING

Running has become hugely popular and is a fantastic form of exercise. I myself have come back to running in the past few years, specifically ultra races in ironman competitions. So to make things a little easier both for first-timers and experienced runners. I thought I would put together a quick reference guide to give you lots of information on running in a simple way! This A–Z has lots of snippets of information that will be a big help to you.

Asics: These are my favourite brand of runners. I have been using the GEL-Kayanos for many years now and I have put the fact that I've had few injuries down to the fact that I change my runners every few months. No matter what type of runner you use, make sure you get some gait analysis done before you buy. You can get this done in Elverys stores across the country and in other stores, such as Amphibian King. A gait analysis will ensure that you get the right runners for your foot type and the best of all is that it's free of charge, so you have nothing to lose.

Blisters: To be avoided. Seam-free socks and properly fitted running shoes will help, and if you still find you're prone to them, try applying Vaseline on those areas before you go out – it will help prevent them from forming.

Cartilage: This is the shock-absorbent tissue in your knees that prevents the bones from rubbing together. It's very important to keep your cartilage in as good condition as possible, and products such as Udo's Oil and Glucosamine Chondroitin will help to ensure that your knees stay in the best possible condition, along with the regular changing of your runners – every four to six months.

Dri-Fit: This is one of any athlete's best friends. Clothing that will help keep you as dry as possible, that works to eliminate the sweat and keep you comfortable; all sports brands use some form of Dri-Fit fabric. The golden rule is to avoid cotton clothing as this holds on to water, becomes heavy and uncomfortable and can increase the risk of chafing or blisters.

Energy drinks: These are overused, over-promoted and to be avoided. The reality is that if your run is under an hour, there is no reason to use sports drinks or isotonic drinks. While they may quench your thirst, they really won't make that huge a difference to your running, although there is some research to suggest that they make a difference mentally. Runs that are over an hour do require more fluid and sports drinks can help improve hydration and deliver much-needed sugar into the body for energy.

Fartlek training: Long before the word intervals came along, fartlek training was doing precisely the same thing. This type of training will help you to increase your speed, by training at two different speeds, i.e. one mile fast and one mile slow. They tend to be tougher sessions that really challenge the body to work hard, but the results are worth it!

Gait analysis: Highly recommended when buying any runners. Basically it is an analysis of your feet and how you walk. Some of us walk too much on the outside, or too much on the inside, others walk perfectly in the middle of the foot. Different walks require different types of runners to ensure that you walk evenly across the foot and that's exactly what a gait analysis check is trying to do. It takes five to ten minutes and is worth the wait and is generally free of charge.

Heart-rate monitors: These are watches that measure your heart rate. Your heart rate will tell you how hard the body is working – the benefit being that you can slow down if you see you are overdoing it. A strap that's placed across your chest is what does all the measuring. It's painless, effective and may help you to stop from hitting the wall in your next marathon!

Insoles: If you develop shin splints or knee injuries, you may be recommended to buy new insoles, especially if you have fallen arches in your feet. Be careful when using them, ease into it slowly.

Jogging: I haven't specifically referred to jogging as part of the BTBW Cardio Plan, but this is what you naturally do when you begin to run. It is like a stepping stone from walking to running. As your fitness improves, you'll be running more than jogging.

Kilometre: Each mile you run is equal to 1.6 kilometres.

Little by little: The best fitness gains are made this way. Aim to increase your running distances in small increments – as the plans here outline. Aside from being steady and sustainable – the BTBW way – this also helps prevent injury and strains.

Mountains: One of the best and most fun ways to improve your road running is to head for the hills and get running in the mountains. There is a mountain-running association that have races all year round, it will build calf and leg power that you previously thought unachievable. When you come back to race on the roads, you will see just how much faster you have become.

Nutrition: People starting off at running often ask if they need to bring fluids/energy foods on their run. The short answer is no. Not unless you are running for over an hour. So don't overcomplicate things for yourself – but do make sure you are properly hydrated setting out on your run, and have eaten a proper BTBW Food Plan meal earlier so as to avoid sharp drops in blood sugar.

Overtraining: This means you are pushing your body too hard. Symptoms such as tiredness, lack of appetite, high heart rates, illness and being in bad form are all indicators of overtraining. The biggest indicator is if you go out for an easy session and it feels extremely hard. If this happens, then simply head for home as quickly as possible, put your feet up and recover. Rest is the best way to recover.

Pacing: If doing a slow interval, avoid speeding up – wait until your fast interval for that. And vice versa – keep up the pace in your fast interval and avoid slowing down. Pacing yourself is an important cornerstone of running.

Quality, not quantity: Don't just run for the sake of getting the miles in, aim to get quality runs in, where you are getting great benefits from the run as opposed to just running for the sake of it. If your body is tired, then get some rest rather than going for a run, it will make all the difference!

Recovery: You have two important times at the end of a run. The first 20 minutes is when you need to get simple carbs into the system. A sports drink or Yazoo will be perfect as they contain the correct ratio of protein to carbs which is 1:4. The second 20 minutes is where you need to get real food into the body, a meal of protein and some carbohydrates would be perfect.

Sat nav: Ok, it may not be sat nav, but GPS watches like the Garmin range will track your speed, time, calories, heart rate, distance and route, using satellite technology. These help to ensure that you're not running too fast, and you can log all your runs on the Garmin website too. I would be lost without mine!

Time: Regardless of whether it's fast walking or running (or whatever the form of exercise), you should aim to time your session. Then when you repeat the session try to go farther in the same time. It means that you will push your body harder, and reap the rewards.

Uplift: Don't forget that all-important sports bra, to support your back and minimise discomfort.

Variation: Aim to vary your running routes as much as you can; the body will adapt more when running different routes, so change your routes as often as possible!

Watches: As your fitness improves, a GPS/heart-rate monitor watch can be an important tool. These types of watches analyse how hard you are working, so help you to set goals and push yourself. GPS watches will even give you your speed and distance for your workouts, ensuring that you really are getting the most out of the session.

Wet gear: Something no runner should do without. Make sure you have at least one rain jacket and one pair of leggings for running throughout the winter months.

Xcountry running: If you are getting a little bored of running on the roads, then why not take it off road and try some cross country running, it will really challenge your legs and lungs and can often put the fun back into running again!

Yazoo: One of my favourite post-running recovery products. These drinks are low in fat and high in carbs with some protein thrown in for good measure. They are good value and you can keep them in the car or at home so as soon as you are finished you can start the recovery process straight away.

Zumo: If you find you sweat a lot during your run or find that you have salty taste in your mouth after a session, then these electrolyte-based tablets can help you to recover very quickly. Most people won't need them but if you do, these are great to use.

APPENDIX 2:
THE A–Z OF WEIGHT LOSS

Absolutely no more excuses: You are sick and tired of falling off the weight-loss wagon – this time it will be for real, for good and without the quick-fix diet solution. Are you ready?

Believe: Forget about the past – it has no place here. If you tell yourself you can't do it, there's a good chance you will prove yourself right. So why not tell yourself you *can* do it – and prove yourself right the best way. Believe. Then keep believing.

Cardiovascular workouts: An essential part of any fitness plan. Your cardiovascular workouts are anything that gets your heart rate up, such as walking, swimming, running, cycling and dancing. They will burn calories, increase your fitness levels, help to firm up the body and help raise your metabolic rate.

DOMS or delayed onset muscle soreness: This explains why you sometimes get pain two days after a tough workout. It is a symptom of muscle damage that occurs during your training; the pain will increase if you work too hard too soon, so exercise caution when you are starting any training.

Epsom salts: One of the greatest and cheapest ways to alleviate pain caused by training. Pick up a tub in your local chemist, add the salts to a hot bath and jump in for 30 minutes or so, this will prevent a lot of the stiffness and get you ready for your next session.

Fat loss: Each 1 pound of fat contains 3,500 calories and that's what you need to aim for through changing your diet and training to lose fat. A lot of the weight loss can be fluid initially.

Garmin: If you are running or cycling as part of your training, I can't recommend a Garmin watch enough. Giving you information about your heart rate, speed, pace, calories and other feedback, it will help you not only to track your workouts, but also to work harder in your sessions, helping to burn more calories and get better results.

Heart rate: Your body can burn different fuel depending on how hard you are working; certain heart-rate zones will help you to burn more fat, depending on the type of training you are doing. Heart-rate monitors are on many machines, but often inaccurate – a heart-rate monitor watch will be much more accurate and they start at fifty euro.

Interval training: One of the best ways to ensure that you are maximising your training time. Intervals apply to any sport, consisting of two speeds, fast and slow. As you get fitter, you reduce the amount of time in the slow zone and increase the amount of time in the fast zone. Intervals help your body to burn more fat in less time – they can be tough, but extremely effective.

Joints: We all have a different genetic make-up. Your joint mobility affects the range of movement that you can achieve in an exercise. While some can do deep squats, other people can't, the general rule of thumb is to go as far as you feel comfortable. If you find that you have joint problems, try to add some glucosamine into your diet; these come in tablet and liquid form, just ensure that they come with chondroitin, as this will help the absorption.

Ketosis: Ketosis is the key behind many quick-fix diets on the market, where your protein levels are increased, triggering the body to use its own fat stores for fuel. It will give you rapid weight loss, but it will also give you bad breath, hard skin and possibly kidney problems.

Love handles: Forget the hundreds of sit-ups or heavy side bends, the only way to get rid of your love handles is a good diet, hard cardiovascular training and full-body resistance training. This combination will yield the quickest and best results.

Mustard and spices: A great way to naturally increase your metabolic rate is to spice up your food as hot as you can, using chilies, mustard and anything else that you like – a great way to help accelerate your weight loss.

New sports: We live in a country surrounded by fantastic amenities, so why not get out there and try them? From rock climbing to surfing, hill walking to mountain biking, there is a sport out there for everyone, so why not give it a go, you never know, you might just enjoy it.

Overtraining: If you push your body too hard, you can overtrain. Symptoms include irritability, loss of appetite, insomnia and soreness after an easy session. If you overtrain, you need to rest up and allow the body to recover; if you continue to get sore after an easy session, then rest for longer until you don't.

Personal trainers: We will help you to achieve your goals. Shop around to ensure you get a trainer that suits you best. They should advise you on nutrition and motivation, helping to set goals. There are hundreds across the country, using different methods but working towards the same goal. Different trainers will have different body types that they will train towards, producing a certain shape. Ensure that it is the type that you want.

Quality: It is no use just doing a session for the fun of it. If your body is very tired, then take the session off. You are aiming to get quality sessions, not quantity. You should finish each session feeling that you have given your best in that session.

Rest: Often overlooked, your body needs rest! No matter how you are training to lose weight, you must ensure that you are taking at least one day per week to put your feet up and let your body recover. Rest will help you to avoid injury and actually improve the results that you get.

Spot reduction: Alas, I am afraid it can't be done. You can't just reduce one area of the body on its own, no matter what any machine or advert will tell you. Your body needs to work as a whole, to get the best results. Aim to do exercise for all the body parts, and the body will evenly tone where it needs to.

Tunes: You will train harder with music, your subconscious adapting to the beat of the song, so pick up a dance CD and pop it on your mp3 player, to help you get the best out of your workouts.

Udo's Oil: One of my favourite products for overall health, Udo's Oil delivers a balanced 2:1:1 ratio of omega-3 to omega-6 and omega-9 essential fatty acids (EFAs) which are essential for all-round health in the body and the body can't produce them. They also come in tablet form, which can be easier to take.

Vibro plates: This is quite a popular weight-loss method, but I must say I have never been a great fan of it. For rehabilitation maybe, but for weight loss and getting results, I feel that there are certainly better ways. If you are going to use them, ensure that you get good instruction, and at the slightest sign of back pain stop straight away.

Walking: I am a huge fan of walking to get results. It's free, accessible and if done properly will yield results. Aim to walk at four miles per hour.

Xenadrine: One of the most popular fat burners on the market – my advice is to avoid it in favour of fresh, great-tasting low-GI food.

Your friends: For best results, surround yourself with positive people – but think twice before you tell everyone around you your plans. You can do without any negativity, so only confide in people you can rely on to support and sustain you on the way.

Zumba: This is currently one of the biggest trends in global fitness. Highly recommended, it's a fun, healthy way to get fit and gets the cardiovascular system working hard. Just ensure that you are also making changes to your diet, to help you get the best results.

> ### A NOTE OF CAUTION:
> Before starting this or any exercise programme, you should always consult your GP to ensure that it is safe for you to exercise. If you have any injuries prior to starting, please visit your local physiotherapist for advice. If you feel sick, dizzy or nauseous at any stage, stop exercising straight away. Ensure you are drinking plenty of water while exercising. Treatment for any injuries should always follow the RICE technique, which stands for rest, ice, compression and elevation.

FITNESS MYTHS

Sit-ups will flatten your stomach: Totally untrue. We all have six-packs but it's the fat that covers them that makes all the difference. I am afraid sit-ups will do relatively little for the fat around your waistline; if anything, too many sit-ups can actually make your waist thicker.

Weights make you bulky: Another fantastic myth. Weights will tone and firm up the muscle, speed up your metabolism and increase your

BMR (basal metabolic rate). They will not make you muscular like Arnold Schwarzenegger. Many people lose weight but stay soft, as their body hasn't toned up.

Cardio alone will get you to your target weight: Cardiovascular workouts such as running, cycling and swimming will help you lose weight, as you burn more calories, but ideally you should combine your cardio workouts with some resistance workouts for the best and quickest results.

Not eating breakfast speeds up your metabolism: By not eating breakfast you actually slow down your metabolism and your weight loss. Never good! Your breakfast is the most important meal of the day, skip it at your peril!

Spinning will make your legs bigger: Controversial one this one, myself and many other trainers believe that by doing too much spinning, your legs can certainly get thicker and more muscular. One spin session a week won't do you any harm; combined as part of an overall plan, it can actually work quite well, but certainly don't overdo it.

WEBSITES OF INTEREST

www.runireland.com

www.henrys.ie

www.wheelworxbikes.com

www.irishfit.eu

www.activeeurope.com

www.mapmyrun.com

www.imra.ie

www.runkeeper.com

www.jellyfishsurfco.com

www.macnallyopticians.com

www.medicosmeticcentre.com

www.coillte.ie

www.isasurf.ie

www.surfcoachireland.com

www.trekbikes.com

www.triathlonireland.com

www.garmin.com

www.magicseaweed.com

www.underarmour.com

www.asics.com

www.runnersworld.com

www.henryfitnesscentre.com

www.karlhenry.ie

APPENDIX 3: RUNNING PLANS

5-KILOMETRE RUN TRAINING PLAN

Below is my favourite 5K training plan that will get you ready for a 5K race in just six weeks. It will get you to the start line fit and ready to race. The important thing to remember is just to take it at your own pace, get your four sessions done each week and don't try to overdo it!

Week 1 training

- Walk for 3 minutes, jog for 1 minute. Repeat 4 times.

- Walk for 3 minutes, jog for 1 minute 30 seconds. Repeat 4 times.

- Walk for 3 minutes, jog for 1 minute 30 seconds. Repeat 4 times.

- 30-minute fast walk.

Week 2 training

- Walk for 2 minutes, run for 1 minute 30 seconds. Repeat 6 times.

- Walk for 2 minutes, run for 2 minutes. Repeat 4 times.

- Walk for 2 minutes, run for 2 minutes. Repeat 5 times.

- 30-minute fast walk.

Week 3 training

- Walk for 2 minutes, run for 2 minutes 30 seconds. Repeat 6 times.

- Walk for 2 minutes, run for 3 minutes. Repeat 4 times.

- Walk for 2 minutes, run for 3 minutes. Repeat 5 times.

- 45-minute fast walk.

Week 4 training

- Walk for 2 minutes, run for 3 minutes. Repeat 6 times.

- Walk for 2 minutes, run for 3 minutes 30 seconds. Repeat 5 times.

- Walk for 2 minutes, run for 4 minutes. Repeat 5 times.

- 1-hour fast walk.

Week 5 training

- Walk for 1 minute 30 seconds, run for 4 minutes. Repeat 6 times.

- Walk for 1 minute 30 seconds, run for 4 minutes. Repeat 6 times.

- Walk for 1 minute 30 seconds, run for 4 minutes 30 seconds. Repeat 5 times.

- 45-minute fast walk.

Week 6 training

- Walk for 1 minute, run for 4 minutes. Repeat 5 times.

- Walk for 1 minute, run for 4 minutes. Repeat 4 times.

- Walk for 1 minute, run for 4 minutes. Repeat 2 times.

- Race or twenty minute fast walk.

10-KILOMETRE RUN TRAINING PLAN

Now that you have conquered the 5K distance you may fancy a 10K and the good news is that with a little extra training, you will be well able to achieve your 10K dreams. It is such a fantastic distance that you will enjoy it so much! This plan is based on four runs a week and one strength and stretching session.

The plan below is based on ten weeks' training and the numbers are all in miles. You will notice a rest day in the plan, which is essential to let the body recover from the running. If you feel over-